T0321081

Arrhythmic and Vascular Complications of Coronavirus Disease 2019 (COVID-19)

Editors

DOMENICO G. DELLA ROCCA
GIOVANNI B. FORLEO
ANDREA NATALE

CARDIAC ELECTROPHYSIOLOGY CLINICS

www.cardiacEP.theclinics.com

Consulting Editors
RANJAN K. THAKUR
ANDREA NATALE

March 2022 • Volume 14 • Number 1

ELSEVIER

1600 John F. Kennedy Boulevard • Suite 1800 • Philadelphia, Pennsylvania, 19103-2899

http://www.theclinics.com

CARDIAC ELECTROPHYSIOLOGY CLINICS Volume 14, Number 1
March 2022 ISSN 1877-9182, ISBN-13: 978-0-323-98731-8

Editor: Joanna Collett
Developmental Editor: Hannah Almira Lopez

Cardiac Electrophysiology Clinics (ISSN 1877-9182) is published quarterly by Elsevier Inc., 360 Park Avenue South, New York, NY 10010-1710. Months of issue are March, June, September, and December. Subscription prices are $247.00 per year for US individuals, $525.00 per year for US institutions, $259.00 per year for Canadian individuals, $549.00 per year for Canadian institutions, $315.00 per year for international individuals, $549.00 per year for international institutions and $100.00 per year for US, Canadian and international students/residents. To receive student/resident rate, orders must be accompanied by name of affilliated institution, date of term, and the signature of program/residency coordinator on institution letterhead. Orders will be billed at individual rate until proof of status is received. Foreign air speed delivery is included in all Clinics subscription prices. All prices are subject to change without notice. **POST-MASTER: Send address changes to Cardiac Electrophysiology Clinics, Elsevier Health Sciences Division, Subscription Customer Service, 3251 Riverport Lane, Maryland Heights, MO 63043. Customer Service: 1-800-654-2452 (US and Canada). From outside of the US and Canada, call 314-477-8871. Fax: 314-447-8029. E-mail: JournalsCustomer-Service-usa@elsevier.com (for print support); JournalsOnlineSupport-usa@elsevier.com (for online support).**

Reprints. For copies of 100 or more of articles in this publication, please contact the Commercial Reprints Department, Elsevier Inc., 360 Park Avenue South, New York, NY 10010-1710. Tel.: 212-633-3874; Fax: 212-633-3820; E-mail: reprints@elsevier.com.

Cardiac Electrophysiology Clinics is covered in *MEDLINE/PubMed (Index Medicus)*.

Contributors

CONSULTING EDITORS

RANJAN K. THAKUR, MD, MPH, MBA, FHRS
Professor of Medicine and Director, Arrhythmia
Service, Thoracic and Cardiovascular Institute,
Sparrow Health System, Michigan State
University, Lansing, Michigan, USA

ANDREA NATALE, MD, FACC, FHRS
Executive Medical Director, Texas Cardiac
Arrhythmia Institute, St. David's Medical
Center, Austin, Texas, USA; Consulting

Professor, Division of Cardiology, Stanford
University, Palo Alto, California, USA; Adjunct
Professor of Medicine, Heart and Vascular
Center, Case Western Reserve University,
Cleveland, Ohio, USA; Director, Interventional
Electrophysiology, Scripps Clinic, San Diego,
California, USA; Senior Clinical Director, EP
Services, California Pacific Medical Center,
San Francisco, California, USA

EDITORS

DOMENICO G. DELLA ROCCA, MD, PhD
Texas Cardiac Arrhythmia Institute, St. David's
Medical Center, Austin, Texas, USA

GIOVANNI B. FORLEO, MD, PhD
Cardiology Unit, Luigi Sacco University
Hospital, Milan, Italy

ANDREA NATALE, MD, FACC, FHRS
Executive Medical Director, Texas Cardiac
Arrhythmia Institute, St. David's Medical

Center, Austin, Texas, USA; Consulting
Professor, Division of Cardiology, Stanford
University, Palo Alto, California, USA; Adjunct
Professor of Medicine, Heart and Vascular
Center, Case Western Reserve University,
Cleveland, Ohio, USA; Director, Interventional
Electrophysiology, Scripps Clinic, San Diego,
California, USA; Senior Clinical Director, EP
Services, California Pacific Medical Center,
San Francisco, California, USA

AUTHORS

SURYA KIRAN AEDMA, MD
Department of Medicine, Carle Foundation
Hospital, Urbana, Illinois, USA; HCA Midwest
Health, Overland Park, Kansas, USA

ADNAN AHMED, MD
Kansas City Heart Rhythm Institute, HCA
Midwest Health, Overland Park, Kansas,
USA

AMIN AL-AHMAD, MD
Texas Cardiac Arrhythmia Institute, St. David's
Medical Center, Austin, Texas, USA

MARIA ALFARANO, MD
Department of Cardiovascular/Respiratory
Diseases, Nephrology, Anesthesiology, and

Geriatric Sciences, Policlinico Umberto I,
Sapienza University of Rome, Rome, Italy

ISABELLA ALVIZ, MD
Montefiore Medical Center, Albert Einstein
College of Medicine, Bronx, New York, USA

ROBERTO AROSIO, MD
Cardiology Unit, Luigi Sacco University
Hospital, Milan, Italy

FEDERICO BALLATORE, MD
Department of Cardiovascular/Respiratory
Diseases, Nephrology, Anesthesiology, and
Geriatric Sciences, Policlinico Umberto I,
Sapienza University of Rome, Rome, Italy

ALBERTO BAROSI, MD
Cardiology Unit, Luigi Sacco University
Hospital, Milan, Italy

MOHAMED BASSIOUNY, MD
Texas Cardiac Arrhythmia Institute, St. David's
Medical Center, Austin, Texas, USA

LUCA BERGAMASCHI, MD
Cardiology Unit, Luigi Sacco University
Hospital, Milan, Italy

ALESSIA BERNARDINI, MD
Department of Cardiovascular/Respiratory
Diseases, Nephrology, Anesthesiology, and
Geriatric Sciences, Policlinico Umberto I,
Sapienza University of Rome, Rome, Italy

FEDERICO BERNARDINI, MD
Department of Cardiovascular/Respiratory
Diseases, Nephrology, Anesthesiology, and
Geriatric Sciences, Policlinico Umberto I,
Sapienza University of Rome, Rome, Italy

GIUSEPPE BIONDI-ZOCCAI, MD
MStat, Division of Cardiology, Santa Maria
Goretti Hospital, Department of Medical-
Surgical Sciences and Biotechnologies,
Sapienza University, Latina, Italy; Mediterranea
Cardiocentro, Naples, Italy

CHIARA BUCCIARELLI-DUCCI, MD, PhD
Brompton and Harefield Hospitals, Guys and
St Thomas NHS Trust and King's College,
London, United Kingdom

J. DAVID BURKHARDT, MD
Texas Cardiac Arrhythmia Institute, St. David's
Medical Center, Austin, Texas, USA

MARIA PAOLA CANALE, MD
Department of Systems Medicine, University of
Rome Tor Vergata, Center for Atherosclerosis,
Policlinico Tor Vergata, Rome, Italy

RISHI CHARATE, MD
Kansas City Heart Rhythm Institute, HCA
Midwest Health, Overland Park, Kansas, USA

CRISTINA CHIMENTI, MD, PhD
Department of Cardiovascular/Respiratory
Diseases, Nephrology, Anesthesiology, and
Geriatric Sciences, Policlinico Umberto I,
Sapienza University of Rome, Cellular and

Molecular Cardiology Lab, IRCCS L.
Spallanzani, Rome, Italy

GAETANO CHIRICOLO, MD
Division of Cardiology, "Tor Vergata" University
Hospital, Department of Biomedicine and
Prevention, "Tor Vergata" University of Rome,
Rome, Italy

DONATELLO CIRONE, MPH
Azienda Ospedaliero-Universitaria Careggi,
Florence, Italy

FRANCESCA CONWAY, MD
Msc Candidate, London School of Hygiene and
Tropical Medicine, London, United Kingdom

IGNAZIO CUSMANO, MD
Cardiology Unit, Luigi Sacco University
Hospital, Milan, Italy

FRANCESCO DE FELICE, MD
Division of Cardiology, San Camillo Hospital,
Rome, Italy

ESTEFANIA DE GARATE, MD
Bristol Heart Institute, University Hospitals
Bristol and Weston NHS Trust and University of
Bristol, Bristol, United Kingdom

ARMANDO DEL PRETE, MD
Division of Cardiology, Santa Maria Goretti
Hospital, Latina, Italy; Department of Systems
Medicine, University of Rome "Tor Vergata,"
Rome, Italy

DOMENICO G. DELLA ROCCA, MD, PhD
Texas Cardiac Arrhythmia Institute, St. David's
Medical Center, Austin, Texas, USA

LUIGI DI BIASE, MD, PhD, FACC, FHRS
Section Head, Electrophysiology, Director,
Arrhythmia Services, Professor, Department
of Medicine, Montefiore Medical Center,
Albert Einstein College of Medicine, Bronx,
New York, USA; Texas Cardiac Arrhythmia
Institute at St. David's Medical Center, Austin,
Texas, USA

MARTINA DI IORIO, MD
Department of Cardiovascular/Respiratory
Diseases, Nephrology, Anesthesiology, and
Geriatric Sciences, Policlinico Umberto I,
Sapienza University of Rome, Rome, Italy

LUCA DI LULLO, MD, PhD
Department of Nephrology and Dialysis, L. Parodi - Delfino Hospital, Colleferro, Roma, Italy

JUAN CARLOS DIAZ, MD
Clinica Las Americas, Medellin, Colombia

FRANCESCO FEDELE, MD
Department of Cardiovascular/Respiratory Diseases, Nephrology, Anesthesiology, and Geriatric Sciences, Policlinico Umberto I, Sapienza University of Rome, Rome, Italy

MASSIMO FEDERICI, MD
Department of Systems Medicine, University of Rome Tor Vergata, Center for Atherosclerosis, Policlinico Tor Vergata, Rome, Italy

GIOVANNI B. FORLEO, MD, PhD
Cardiology Unit, Luigi Sacco University Hospital, Milan, Italy

FEDELE FRANCESCO, MD
Department of Cardiovascular/Respiratory Diseases, Nephrology, Anesthesiology, and Geriatric Sciences, Policlinico Umberto I, Sapienza University of Rome, Rome, Italy

ANDREA FRUSTACI, MD
Department of Cardiovascular/Respiratory Diseases, Nephrology, Anesthesiology, and Geriatric Sciences, Policlinico Umberto I, Sapienza University of Rome, Cellular and Molecular Cardiology Lab, IRCCS L. Spallanzani, Rome, Italy

MOHAMED GABR, MD
Montefiore Medical Center, Albert Einstein College of Medicine, Bronx, New York, USA

G. JOSEPH GALLINGHOUSE, MD
Texas Cardiac Arrhythmia Institute, St. David's Medical Center, Austin, Texas, USA

MARIA T. GAMERO, MD
Montefiore Medical Center, Albert Einstein College of Medicine, Bronx, New York, USA

URIEL GARCIA, BS
Universidad Anahuac, Mexico City, Mexico

ALESSIO GASPERETTI, MD
Cardiology Unit, Luigi Sacco University Hospital, Milan, Italy; Division of Cardiology, Johns Hopkins University, Baltimore, Maryland, USA

ELISA GHERBESI, MD
Cardiology Unit, Luigi Sacco University Hospital, Milan, Italy

CAROLA GIANNI, MD, PhD
Texas Cardiac Arrhythmia Institute, St. David's Medical Center, Austin, Texas, USA

GIUSEPPE GIUNTA, MD
Department of Cardiovascular/Respiratory Diseases, Nephrology, Anesthesiology, and Geriatric Sciences, Policlinico Umberto I, Sapienza University of Rome, Rome, Italy

RAKESH GOPINATHANNAIR, MD
Kansas City Heart Rhythm Institute, HCA Midwest Health, Overland Park, Kansas, USA

RODNEY P. HORTON, MD
Texas Cardiac Arrhythmia Institute, St. David's Medical Center, Austin, Texas, USA

DUDLEY J. PENNELL, MD
Royal Brompton and Harefield Hospitals, Guys and St Thomas NHS Trust and Imperial College London, London, United Kingdom

DHANUNJAYA LAKKIREDDY, MD, FACC, FHRS
Executive Medical Director, Kansas City Heart Rhythm Institute, HCA Midwest Health, Overland Park, Kansas, USA; Professor of Medicine, University of Missouri-Columbia, Columbia, Missouri, USA

CARLO LAVALLE, MD
Department of Cardiovascular/Respiratory Diseases, Nephrology, Anesthesiology, and Geriatric Sciences, Policlinico Umberto I, Sapienza University of Rome, Rome, Italy

DALGISIO LECIS, MD
Division of Cardiology, "Tor Vergata" University Hospital, Rome, Italy

KATE LIANG, MBBCh
Bristol Heart Institute, University Hospitals Bristol and Weston NHS Trust and University of Bristol, Bristol, United Kingdom

AUNG LIN, MD
Montefiore Medical Center, Albert Einstein College of Medicine, Bronx, New York USA

BRYAN MACDONALD, MD
Texas Cardiac Arrhythmia Institute, St. David's
Medical Center, Austin, Texas, USA

MICHELE MAGNOCAVALLO, MD
Texas Cardiac Arrhythmia Institute, St. David's
Medical Center, Austin, Texas, USA;
Department of Cardiovascular/Respiratory
Diseases, Nephrology, Anesthesiology, and
Geriatric Sciences, Policlinico Umberto I,
Sapienza University of Rome, Rome, Italy

MARCO VALERIO MARIANI, MD
Department of Cardiovascular/Respiratory
Diseases, Nephrology, Anesthesiology, and
Geriatric Sciences, Policlinico Umberto I,
Sapienza University of Rome, Rome, Italy

EUGENIO MARTELLI, MD
Department of General and Specialist Surgery
"P. Stefanini", Sapienza University of Rome,
Rome, Italy; Division of Vascular Surgery, S.
Anna and S. Sebastiano Hospital, Caserta,
Italy

EUGENIO MARTUSCELLI, MD
Division of Cardiology, "Tor Vergata" University
Hospital, Department of Biomedicine and
Prevention, "Tor Vergata" University of Rome,
Rome, Italy

GIANLUCA MASSARO, MD
Division of Cardiology, "Tor Vergata" University
Hospital, Rome, Italy

JOSE MATIAS, MD
Montefiore Medical Center, Albert Einstein
College of Medicine, Bronx, New York, USA

ANGEL MAYEDO, MD
Texas Cardiac Arrhythmia Institute, St. David's
Medical Center, Austin, Texas, USA

MARIA CHIARA MEI, MD
Department of Cardiovascular/Respiratory
Diseases, Nephrology, Anesthesiology, and
Geriatric Sciences, Policlinico Umberto I,
Sapienza University of Rome, Rome, Italy

ROSSELLA MENGHINI, PhD
Department of Systems Medicine, University of
Rome Tor Vergata, Rome, Italy

FABIO MIRALDI, MD
Department of Cardiovascular/Respiratory
Diseases, Nephrology, Anesthesiology, and
Geriatric Sciences, Policlinico Umberto I,
Sapienza University of Rome, Rome, Italy

GIANFRANCO MITACCHIONE, MD, PhD
Cardiology Unit, Luigi Sacco University
Hospital, Milan, Italy

SANGHAMITRA MOHANTY, MD, MS
Texas Cardiac Arrhythmia Institute, St. David's
Medical Center, Austin, Texas, USA

CARMINE MUSTO, MD, PhD
Division of Cardiology, San Camillo Hospital,
Rome, Italy

ELENI NAKOU, MD, PhD
CMR Unit, Royal Brompton and Harefield
Hospitals, Guys and St Thomas NHS
Foundation Trust, Sydney Street, London,
United Kingdom

ANDREA NATALE, MD, FACC, FHRS
Executive Medical Director, Texas Cardiac
Arrhythmia Institute, St. David's Medical
Center, Austin, Texas, USA; Consulting
Professor, Division of Cardiology, Stanford
University, Palo Alto, California, USA; Adjunct
Professor of Medicine, Heart and Vascular
Center, Case Western Reserve University,
Cleveland, Ohio, USA; Director, Interventional
Electrophysiology, Scripps Clinic, San Diego,
California, USA; Senior Clinical Director, EP
Services, California Pacific Medical Center,
San Francisco, California, USA

MARCO PICICHÈ, MD
Department of Cardiac Surgery, San Bortolo
Hospital, Vicenza, Italy

AGOSTINO PIRO, MD
Department of Cardiovascular/Respiratory
Diseases, Nephrology, Anesthesiology, and
Geriatric Sciences, Policlinico Umberto I,
Sapienza University of Rome, Rome, Italy

NAGA VENKATA K. POTHINENI, MD
Kansas City Heart Rhythm Institute, HCA
Midwest Health, Overland Park, Kansas, USA;
Section of Electrophysiology, Division of

Cardiovascular Medicine, University of
Pennsylvania, Philadelphia, Pennsylvania, USA

SUTOPA PURKAYASTHA, MD
Montefiore Medical Center, Albert Einstein
College of Medicine, Bronx, New York, USA

RAFFAELE QUAGLIONE, MD
Department of Cardiovascular/Respiratory
Diseases, Nephrology, Anesthesiology, and
Geriatric Sciences, Policlinico Umberto I,
Sapienza University of Rome, Rome, Italy

OLGA REYNBAKH, MD
Montefiore Medical Center, Albert Einstein
College of Medicine, Bronx, New York, USA

JORGE ROMERO, MD, FACC, FHRS
Montefiore Medical Center, Albert Einstein
College of Medicine, Bronx, New York, USA

JAVIER E. SANCHEZ, MD
Texas Cardiac Arrhythmia Institute, St. David's
Medical Center, Austin, Texas, USA

GIUSEPPE MASSIMO SANGIORGI, MD
Division of Cardiology, "Tor Vergata" University
Hospital, Department of Biomedicine and
Prevention, "Tor Vergata" University of Rome,
Rome, Italy

PASQUALE SANTANGELI, MD, PhD
Section of Electrophysiology, Division of
Cardiovascular Medicine, University of
Pennsylvania, Philadelphia, Pennsylvania, USA

MARCO SCHIAVONE, MD
Cardiology Unit, Luigi Sacco University
Hospital, Milan, Italy

PAOLO SEVERINO, MD, PhD
Department of Cardiovascular/Respiratory
Diseases, Nephrology, Anesthesiology, and
Geriatric Sciences, Policlinico Umberto I,
Sapienza University of Rome, Rome, Italy

SAISHISHIR SHETTY, DPharm, MHI
Texas Cardiac Arrhythmia Institute, St. David's
Medical Center, Austin, Texas, USA

NICOLA TARANTINO, MD
Montefiore Medical Center, Bronx, New York,
USA

PATRICK UDENYI, BS
University of California, Berkeley, Berkeley,
California, USA

ALEJANDRO VELASCO, MD
Montefiore Medical Center, Albert Einstein
College of Medicine, Bronx, New York,
USA

FRANCESCO VERSACI, MD
Division of Cardiology, Santa Maria Goretti
Hospital, Latina, Italy

GIAMPAOLO VETTA, MD
Department of Cardiovascular/Respiratory
Diseases, Nephrology, Anesthesiology, and
Geriatric Sciences, Policlinico Umberto I,
Sapienza University of Rome, Rome,
Italy

MAURIZIO VIECCA, MD
Cardiology Unit, Luigi Sacco University
Hospital, Milan, Italy

CARMINE DARIO VIZZA, MD
Department of Cardiovascular/Respiratory
Diseases, Nephrology, Anesthesiology, and
Geriatric Sciences, Policlinico Umberto I,
Sapienza University of Rome, Rome, Italy

MATTHEW WILLIAMS, MBChB BSc
Bristol Heart Institute, University Hospitals
Bristol and Weston NHS Trust and University of
Bristol, Bristol, United Kingdom

WILLIAM ZAGRODZKY, BS
Texas Cardiac Arrhythmia Institute, St. David's
Medical Center, Austin, Texas, USA

FENGWEI ZOU, MD
Montefiore Medical Center, Albert Einstein
College of Medicine, Bronx, New York
USA

Contents

> COVID-19 mainly affects the respiratory system but has been correlated with cardio-vascular manifestations such as myocarditis, heart failure, acute coronary syn-dromes, and arrhythmias. Cardiac arrhythmias are the second most frequent complication affecting about 30% of patients. Several mechanisms may lead to an increased risk of cardiac arrhythmias during COVID-19 infection, ranging from direct myocardial damage to extracardiac involvement. The aim of this review is to describe the role of COVID-19 in the pathogenesis of cardiac arrhythmias and provide a comprehensive guidance for their monitoring and management.

> We review the current data on epidemiology, the clinical significance, the patho-physiologic mechanisms, and the treatment of VAs in the setting of COVID-19. VAs prevail in 0.15% to 8% of hospitalized patients, but only sustained and rapid tachyarrhythmias are purportedly associated with a significant increase in mortal-ity. Multiple factors can elicit VAs, which are ultimately deemed to be a marker of severe systemic disease rather than a distinct cardiac condition. Even though the electrophysiologist plays a determinant role in the secondary prevention of VAs, a multidisciplinary approach is indispensable for primary prophylaxis and acute management.

> Coronavirus-19 disease (COVID-19) affects more people than previous coronavi-rus infections and has a higher mortality. Higher incidence and mortality can prob-ably be explained by COVID-19 causative agent's greater affinity (about 10–20 times) for angiotensin-converting enzyme 2 (ACE2) receptor compared with other coronaviruses. Here, the authors first summarize clinical manifestations, then pre-sent symptoms of COVID-19 and the pathophysiological mechanisms underlying specific organ/system disease. The worse clinical outcome observed in COVID-19 patients with diabetes may be in part related to the increased ADAM17 activity and its unbalanced interplay with ACE2. Therefore, strategies aimed to inhibit ADAM17 activity may be explored to develop new effective therapeutic approaches.

> Severe acute respiratory syndrome coronavirus-2 can affect the cardiovascular system yielding a wide range of complications, including acute myocardial injury. The myocardium can be damaged by direct viral invasion or indirect mechanisms, sustained by systemic inflammation, immune-mediated response, and dysregulation of the renin-angiotensin system. Myocardial injury affects about one-quarter of patients with COVID-19, can manifest even in the absence of previous cardiovascular disease, and is associated to higher mortality rates and long-term sequelae. This review describes the pathophysiological mechanisms of myocardial injury and infarction and discusses the main clinical outcomes and diagnostic challenges associated with myocardial damage during COVID-19.

> COVID-19 is an acute respiratory disease of viral origin caused by SARS-CoV-2. This disease is associated with a hypercoagulable state resulting in arterial and venous thrombotic events. The latter are more frequent, especially in patients who develop a severe form of the disease and are associated with an increased mortality rate. It is therefore essential to identify patients at higher risk to initiate antithrombotic therapy. Hospitalized patients treated with treatment dose of anticoagulants had better outcomes than those treated with prophylactic dose. However, several trials are ongoing to better define the therapeutic and prevention strategies for this insidious complication.

> The clinical manifestations of COVID-19 are widely variable and may involve several districts. Although the clinical course is mostly characterized by respiratory involvement, up to 30% of hospitalized patients have evidence of myocardial injury due to acute coronary syndrome, cardiac arrhythmias, myocarditis, and cardiogenic shock. In particular, myocarditis is a well-recognized severe complication of COVID-19 and is associated with fulminant cardiogenic shock and sudden cardiac death. In this article, the authors aim to present a comprehensive review about COVID-19–related myocarditis, including clinical characteristics, diagnostic workup, and management.

> Numerous systemic manifestations, including cardiac involvement in the form of myocardial infarction, myocarditis, and electrocardiographic changes, have been associated with COVID-19. .In this review, the authors describe the

unprecedented health care crisis across the globe. Health care efforts across the world have been diverted to tackling the pandemic since early 2020. Hospitals and health care systems have undertaken major restructuring in an effort to deliver health care to an increasing number of patients affected by COVID-19. Although great focus has been placed on treating those individuals suffering from COVID-19, clinicians must simultaneously balance caring for patients who are not actively infected. In anticipation of an exponential increase in COVID-19 cases, health care systems developed strategies to channel available resources to meet the rapidly rising demands of COVID-19. This change was noticed significantly in the field of invasive cardiology as well. Many cardiac catheterization and electrophysiology (EP) laboratories canceled elective procedures to limit the burden on hospital resources and preserve personal protective equipment (PPE). Major societies published guidance statements delineating patient selection for procedures during the exponential phase of the pandemic growth. Patient care was triaged and those waiting for elective procedures were managed with expectant care or noninvasive approaches to preserve hospital resources and personnel. In the current article, we review the impact of the COVID-19 pandemic and its response to the volume of interventional cardiology (IC) and EP procedures across the world.

During the coronavirus disease 2019 (COVID-19) worldwide pandemic, patients with cardiac implantable electronic device (CIED) refused scheduled follow-up visits because of the risk of infection. In this scenario, different telemedicine strategies have been implemented to ensure continuity of care to CIED patients. Patients can be monitored through dedicated applications, telephone calls, or virtual visits providing easy access to valuable information, such as arrhythmic events, acute decompensation manifestations, and device-related issues, without the need for in-person visits. This review provides a comprehensive description of the many possible applications of telemedicine for CIED patients during the COVID-19 period.

CARDIAC ELECTROPHYSIOLOGY CLINICS

Preface

Arrhythmic and Vascular Complications of Coronavirus Disease 2019

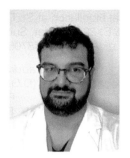

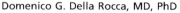

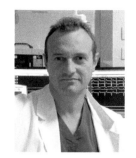

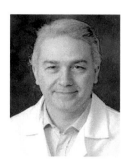

Domenico G. Della Rocca, MD, PhD   Giovanni B. Forleo, MD, PhD   Andrea Natale, MD

Editors

The current coronavirus disease 2019 (COVID-19) pandemic has posed unprecedented challenges for society and health care systems. The outbreak has fueled a global, multidisciplinary research initiative aimed at disclosing the pathophysiologic bases, as well as identifying effective diagnostic and treatment strategies for this disease. This research effort has led to significant discoveries and culminated in the development of effective vaccines against the severe acute respiratory syndrome coronavirus 2 (SARS-CoV-2).

A large body of evidence has suggested that the protean clinical manifestations of SARS-CoV-2 may be explained by a complex pathophysiology, which includes impaired endothelial cell function and microcirculation. Specifically, endothelial activation and dysfunction may alter the integrity of blood vessels and contribute to a procoagulative state, thereby leading to a wide variety of clinical manifestations, which frequently involve the cardiovascular system.

As a result of the impressive numbers of COVID-19 patients requiring hospitalizations, enormous efforts were needed to ensure non-COVID-19 patients could safely and effectively access needed health care. While entire departments were converted to accommodate COVID-19 case surge, the need for new modalities of delivering health care services led to a widespread adoption of digital health solutions (eg, virtual visits, remote monitoring).

This issue of *Cardiac Electrophysiology Clinics* is focused on the prevalence, pathophysiology, diagnosis, and treatment of the arrhythmic and vascular complications of COVID-19.

The first section of six articles is an overview of most common cardiovascular complications of COVID-19. Specifically, articles by Magnocavallo and colleagues and Tarantino and colleagues focus on the prevalence, management, and outcomes of supraventricular and ventricular arrhythmias. The next article, by Paola Canale and colleagues, provides valuable insights into the pathophysiologic bases of SARS-CoV-2-mediated endothelial dysfunction and microvascular injury, which are then discussed (authored by Del Prete and colleagues, Massaro and colleagues, and Chimenti) as a background for specific cardiovascular manifestations (vascular complications, thromboembolism, myocarditis).

The second section of four articles (authored by Romero and colleagues, Barosi and colleagues, Nakou and colleagues, and Schiavone and colleagues) explores the main electrocardiographic and imaging features of COVID-19 and the role of electrocardiography to monitor the proarrhythmic effect of QT prolonging drugs to treat COVID-19.

The last section of this issue (articles authored by Pothineni and Santangeli, Mohanty and colleagues, Ahmed and colleagues, and Magnocavallo and colleagues) focuses on the importance

Card Electrophysiol Clin 14 (2022) xv–xvi
https://doi.org/10.1016/j.ccep.2021.12.012
1877-9182/22/© 2021 Published by Elsevier Inc.

of universal testing strategies to promote workplace safety and on the impact of the pandemic on health care utilization for non-COVID-19 patients, with a spotlight on the widespread adoption of digital health technologies.

We are confident that this issue of *Cardiac Electrophysiology Clinics* will be very useful to health care provides across different specialties, and we wish to thank all the authors for their valuable contributions.

Domenico G. Della Rocca, MD, PhD
Texas Cardiac Arrhythmia Institute
St. David's Medical Center
3000 North IH-35, Suite 720
Austin, TX 78705, USA

Giovanni B. Forleo, MD, PhD
Department of Cardiology
Azienda Ospedaliera-
Universitaria "Luigi Sacco"
Via G.B Grassi, 74
20157 Milan, Italy

Andrea Natale, MD
Texas Cardiac Arrhythmia Institute
Center for Atrial Fibrillation at St. David's
Medical Center, 1015 E. 32nd Street, Suite 516
Austin ,TX 78705, USA

E-mail addresses:
domenicodellarocca@hotmail.it (D.G. Della
Rocca)
forleo@me.com (G.B. Forleo)
dr.natale@gmail.com (A. Natale)

Prevalence, Management, and Outcome of Atrial Fibrillation and Other Supraventricular Arrhythmias in COVID-19 Patients

Michele Magnocavallo, MD[a,b], Giampaolo Vetta, MD[b],
Domenico G. Della Rocca, MD, PhD[a,*], Carola Gianni, MD, PhD[a],
Sanghamitra Mohanty, MD[a], Mohamed Bassiouny, MD[a],
Luca Di Lullo, MD, PhD[c], Armando Del Prete, MD[d], Donatello Cirone, MPH[e],
Carlo Lavalle, MD[b], Cristina Chimenti, MD, PhD[b], Amin Al-Ahmad, MD[a],
J. David Burkhardt, MD[a], G. Joseph Gallinghouse, MD[a],
Javier E. Sanchez, MD[a], Rodney P. Horton, MD[a], Luigi Di Biase, MD, PhD;[a,f],
Andrea Natale, MD[a,g,h]

KEYWORDS

- COVID-19 • Supraventricular arrhythmias • Atrial fibrillation • Catheter ablation • Atrial flutter
- Rhythm control

KEY POINTS

- Supraventricular arrhythmias are common in COVID-19 patients, especially in critically ill.
- Arrhythmias occur after direct viral damage, but also due to systemic involvement.
- Atrial fibrillation represents the most common supraventricular arrhythmias and it is independently associated with in-hospital mortality.
- Supraventricular arrhythmias will be safely treated, minimizing exposure and paying attention to general clinical conditions.

INTRODUCTION

Severe acute respiratory syndrome coronavirus 2 (SARS-COV-2) is the causative agent of coronavirus disease 2019 (COVID-19); it was officially detected for the first time in Wuhan and has spread throughout the world becoming a pandemic.[1,2]

Although COVID-19 causes respiratory symptoms in most patients, several studies showed an extrapulmonary involvement, including the cardiovascular system.[3–5] COVID-19 patients may be affected by myocarditis, thromboembolic events, heart failure and cardiogenic shock, acute coronary syndromes,

M. Magnocavallo and G. Vetta equally contributed to the article.

[a] Texas Cardiac Arrhythmia Institute, St. David's Medical Center, 3000 N. IH-35, Suite 720, Austin, TX 78705, USA; [b] Department of Cardiovascular/Respiratory Diseases, Nephrology, Anesthesiology, and Geriatric Sciences, Policlinico Umberto I, Sapienza University of Rome, Rome, Italy; [c] Department of Nephrology and Dialysis, L. Parodi - Delfino Hospital, Colleferro, Roma, Italy; [d] Division of Cardiology, Santa Maria Goretti Hospital, Latina, Italy; [e] Azienda Ospedaliero-Universitaria Careggi, Florence, Italy; [f] Albert Einstein College of Medicine at Montefiore Hospital, New York, NY, USA; [g] Interventional Electrophysiology, Scripps Clinic, La Jolla, CA, USA; [h] Department of Cardiology, MetroHealth Medical Center, Case Western Reserve University School of Medicine, Cleveland, OH, USA

* Corresponding author. Texas Cardiac Arrhythmia Institute at St. David's Medical Center, 3000 North I-35, Suite 720, Austin, TX 78705.

E-mail address: domenicodellarocca@hotmail.it

Card Electrophysiol Clin 14 (2022) 1–9
https://doi.org/10.1016/j.ccep.2021.10.001
1877-9182/22/© 2021 Elsevier Inc. All rights reserved.

and atrial and ventricular arrhythmias.[6–8] Notably, cardiac arrhythmias occur in 6% to 17% of patients, rising to 44% in patients admitted to the intensive care unit,[9] resulting the second most frequent complication after acute respiratory distress syndrome.[10] Several possible mechanisms lead to an increased risk of cardiac arrhythmias during COVID-19 infection, ranging from direct myocardial injury to extracardiac involvement.[11] Arrhythmias are mainly caused by the hypoxia related to direct viral damage in the lungs, myocarditis, or abnormal inflammatory response and secondarily as a result of myocardial ischemia, myocardial strain, or electrolyte imbalances.[11] As a matter of fact, arrhythmias are not simply caused by the direct effect of COVID-19 infection, but instead are probably the result of a multifactorial condition.[12]

Supraventricular arrhythmias are the most frequent arrhythmias observed in COVID-19 patients and among them, atrial fibrillation (AF) is the most common occurring in about 15% to 30% of them.[13] The presence of AF is associated with increased clinical manifestations of severe COVID-19 and is independently associated with in-hospital mortality, posing a significant burden to patients, physicians, and health care systems globally.[14] The complexity of this clinical condition requires a multifaceted and multidisciplinary approach; thus, we provide a comprehensive guidance for monitoring and management of cardiac arrhythmias in COVID-19 patients.

MECHANISMS OF ARRHYTHMOGENESIS IN COVID-19

COVID-19 infection can lead to an increased risk of cardiac arrhythmias by several pathophysiological mechanisms, which are summarized in **Fig. 1**. These include different types of myocardial injury and extracardiac processes that may exacerbate arrhythmias in patients with a pre-existing propensity.[15]

Hypoxia

The most recurrent COVID-19 manifestation is respiratory involvement, which may progress to acute respiratory distress syndrome. Hypoxia results in anaerobic glycolysis causing a decrease of intracellular pH and electrolyte imbalance, mainly an increase of calcium levels.[16] A higher cytosolic Ca^{2+} concentration alters cellular action potentials and contribute to the development of early and late afterdepolarizations, which are a known trigger for atrial and ventricular arrhythmias.[16] Anaerobiosis also results in an increased potassium concentration and, as a consequence, increased cellular excitability and electrical conduction velocity.[16] In addition, hypoxia reduces electrical coupling and tissue anisotropy via inactivation of connexin-43 in the gap junctions.[17]

Moreover, respiratory failure causes a hyperadrenergic tone, which contributes to the risk of cardiac arrhythmias.[18] Indeed, hypersympathetic activity leads to an amplified calcium influx into cardiomyocytes, resulting in a calcium overload and frequently delayed afterdepolarizations.[19]

Myocarditis

Several findings suggest that SARS-CoV-2 is the causative agent of myocarditis and that myocardium involvement may occur by direct virus infection or through infected alveolar macrophages.[20,21] The virus penetrates the myocardial cell, binding the receptors of the angiotensin-converting enzyme-2 (ACE-2) that will be internalized, leading to a consequent inhibition of angiotensin II degradation.[22,23] The downregulation of myocardial ACE-2 expression is associated with excessive accumulation of angiotensin II, which causes myocardial injury, remodeling, and even adverse cardiac outcomes.[24] Thus, downregulation of ACE-2 in COVID-19 might increase AF vulnerability and its perpetuation.

Another potential mechanism is that virus-activated CD8+ T lymphocytes reach the myocardium and can cause myocardial inflammation, as a result of the release of proinflammatory cytokines and activation of T lymphocytes.[21]

In the acute phase of myocarditis, arrhythmogenesis is caused by cellular damage, ionic imbalance, and gap junction dysfunction due to impaired cardiac connexin expression.[25] In myocarditis, inflammation leads to impaired cellular calcium and potassium homeostasis, producing early and delayed afterdepolarizations and increasing cellular repolarization and conduction time.[25] Prolonged repolarization time leads to triggered activity, whereas coupling with increased conduction time leads to re-entry circuits.[25]

Myocardial Ischemia

Myocardial ischemia in COVID-19 patients could be caused by coronary dysfunction and hyperinflammatory response.[26] The release of cytokines promotes the activation of T lymphocytes and monocytes within a pre-existing atherosclerotic plaque; the resulting histotoxic effect may cause plaque rupture, thereby leading to an acute coronary syndrome. Moreover, the release of the aforementioned cytokines, specifically interleukin (IL)-6, may exert proatherogenic effects, characterized by vascular smooth muscle proliferation, endothelial cell, and platelet activation.[27,28]

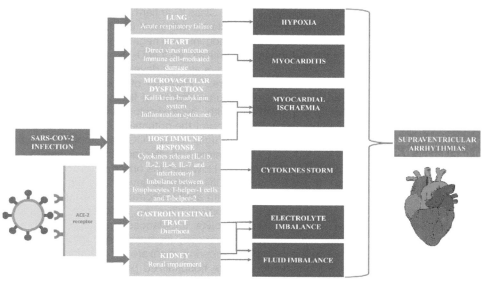

Fig. 1. Potential mechanisms of arrhythmia and COVID-19. IL, interleukin; SARS-CoV-2, severe acute respiratory syndrome coronavirus 2.

Myocardial ischemia can also be caused by microvascular dysfunction due to endothelial impairment.[29,30] Endothelial dysfunction in COVID-19 patients is caused primarily by the downregulation of ACE-2 receptors, triggering the kallikrein-bradykinin system and resulting in increased vascular permeability.[31] Neutrophils and T lymphocytes release inflammatory cytokines and vasoactive molecules increasing endothelial cell contractility and vascular permeability.

Virus-mediated vasculitis is another possible mechanism of microvascular dysfunction because the virus penetrates vascular endothelial cells via ACE-2 receptors, leading to inflammation and apoptosis.[32]

Cytokine Storm

COVID-19 infection causes systemic inflammation and hyperactivation of lymphocytes and monocytes cells, resulting in a cytokine storm (IL-1b, IL-2, IL-6, IL-7, and interferon-γ) and an imbalance between lymphocytes T-helper-1 and T-helper-2 cells.[33] Distinctive cytokines have been shown to induce AF: tumor necrosis factor-α (TNF-α) increases AF vulnerability and exerts direct effects on atrial structural and electrical remodeling[34–36]; TNF-α and IL-1β may impair cardiac contractility, which is a known risk factor for arrhythmogenesis; IL-6 reduces cardiac connexins and promotes electrical remodeling during acute inflammation.[37,38] Furthermore, IL-6, TNF-α, and IL-1 can lead to prolongation of the cardiac action potential due to impairment of K^+ and Ca^{2+} channels.[39]

Electrolyte Imbalance and Fluid Overload

Electrolyte abnormalities are a well-known trigger of arrhythmogenesis.[40] In a study of 416 hospitalized patients with COVID-19 infection, 7.2% of patients had electrolyte disturbances, such as hypokalemia, hypomagnesemia, and hypophosphatemia.[4] In particular, hypokalemia is very frequent in patients with COVID-19, affecting up to 61% of hospitalized patients.[41] These electrolyte imbalances were primarily caused by COVID-19–associated diarrhea and renal impairment.[4] Indeed, in a retrospective study of hospitalized patients with COVID-19 infection, 27% of patients had acute renal failure.[42] In addition, SARS-CoV-2 causes downregulation of ACE-2 receptors and thereby reduces the feedback effects of ACE-2 on the renin-angiotensin-aldosterone system.[41] This leads to increased reabsorption of sodium and water, resulting in increased blood pressure and excretion of potassium. The resulting hypokalemia causes hyperpolarization of the myocardiocytes, predisposing to atrial arrhythmias.[43]

SUPRAVENTRICULAR TACHYCARDIA PREVALENCE AND OUTCOME

Supraventricular arrhythmias are the most frequent arrhythmias among COVID-19 patients.[44,45] In a recent worldwide survey, about 18% of enrolled patients developed any arrhythmias[46]: most of them were supraventricular arrhythmias (81.3%), AF representing the most common (61.5%). In another retrospective study,

166 patients experienced atrial arrhythmias (15.8%) and newly diagnosed atrial arrhythmias occurred in 101 patients (9.6%), corroborating the central role of virus infection in the pathogenesis of cardiac arrhythmias.[14]

Overall, a recent meta-analysis demonstrated that the occurrence of supraventricular arrhythmias was more frequent in critically ill patients (relative risk: 12.1; 95% confidence interval, 8.5–17.3), in particular those treated with invasive mechanical ventilation.[47,48]

The occurrence of supraventricular arrhythmias is associated with worse outcomes. Indeed, hospital admission in the intensive care unit and thromboembolic risk (pulmonary embolism, stroke, or deep vein thrombosis) was higher in COVID-19 patients with atrial arrhythmia than the general population.[49] Therefore, giving the critical conditions of these patients, it is not unexpected that AF should be considered as an independent predictor of 30-day mortality (adjusted odds ratio: 1.93; $P = .007$).[14]

MANAGEMENT OF SUPRAVENTRICULAR ARRHYTHMIAS

The correct management of supraventricular arrhythmias has a central role in COVID-19 patients, especially those hospitalized with more severe forms of the disease and whose outcomes strictly depend on hemodynamic stability. Although there are few studies about the treatment of arrhythmia in COVID-19 patients, it is necessary to take particular attention to the paroxysmal features of arrhythmias, drug-drug interactions, and limitation of exposure.[50,51] Given the overwhelming prevalence of AF and atrial flutter (AFL) in patients with COVID-19, we will focus on the treatment of these arrhythmias.

Rhythm Control

Patients with hemodynamic instability due to new-onset AF and AFL should undergo electrical cardioversion (**Fig. 2**). The choice for electrical cardioversion inevitably involves the need for personnel at bedside, and the possibility of invasive mechanical ventilation, that would increase the development of viral aerosols.[50] Intravenous infusion of amiodarone is recommended for rhythm control in critically ill patients.[51,52] Moreover, we should be aware of the combination of amiodarone with hydroxychloroquine and/or azithromycin, as the benefit of the eventual combination has to be weighed against the arrhythmic risk caused by QT prolongation.[50,53] All interactions between medications for AF and COVID-19 are summarized in **Table 1**.

Class IC antiarrhythmic agents should be administered with great caution because of their arrhythmogenic and negative inotropic effect, especially in critically ill COVID-19 patients, who are prone to or have already developed myocarditis and heart failure.[54] Because of possible increases in plasma concentration of flecainide when co-administered with hydroxychloroquine and lopinavir/ritonavir and/or the potential QT-prolonging effects of these drugs, serial ECG monitoring is recommended before and after initiating drug therapy.

However, the only rhythm control strategy is not sufficient to achieve a long-term benefit in patients with acute respiratory failure, if the other existing comorbidities (eg, hypoxemia, inflammation, electrolyte imbalances, metabolic acidosis, volume overload, increased sympathetic tone, bacterial superinfection) are not properly treated.[50,55] In stable hospitalized patients with AF, antiarrhythmic drugs (such as sotalol, flecainide, amiodarone, and propafenone) should be discontinued and rate control therapy initiated with beta-blockers (or nondihydropyridine calcium channel blockers, unless contraindicated, with or without digoxin) because these drugs represent a safer option when administered in combination with an antiviral therapy.[50] The combination of verapamil with hydroxychloroquine should be avoided because both drugs exert a negative effect on sinoatrial and atrioventricular nodes causing bradycardia and conduction disturbances.[56] Therefore, ECG monitoring for bradycardia and conduction disturbance should be considered. All interactions between medications for AF and COVID-19 are summarized in **Table 1**.

Anticoagulation Therapy

In COVID-19 patients, anticoagulation is prescribed according to the CHA_2DS_2-VASc score.[57] It is important to highlight that some drugs for the treatment of COVID-19 infection have significant interactions with direct oral anticoagulants (DOACs; **Table 1**).[58] In particular, lopinavir and ritonavir may have interactions with cytochrome P450 CYP3A4 and antimalarial drugs through P-glycoprotein inhibition.[59] In these cases, DOACs should be avoided to reduce the risk of bleeding.[60]

In general, DOACs should be favored over vitamin K antagonists (VKAs), given their better safety profile and the standard, international normalized ratio-independent dosing modalities.[61] Indeed, VKAs treatment requires regular monitoring of the international normalized ratio,[62] increasing contact with medical staff, so VKAs should be used preferably only in patients with mechanical prosthetic valves or antiphospholipid syndrome.[62] Heparins have no

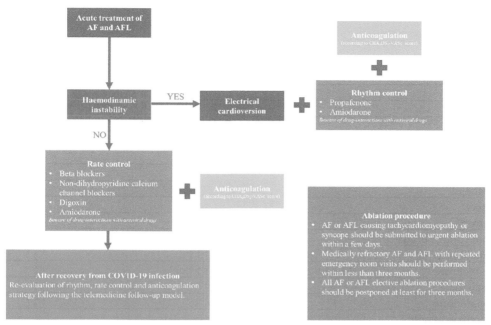

Fig. 2. Acute treatment of AF and AFL in COVID-19 patients. AF, atrial fibrillation; AFL, atrial flutter.

pharmacologic interactions with drugs for the treatment of COVID-19, making them a safe alternative to oral anticoagulants. Moreover, heparin could provide an anti-inflammatory role in addition to its anticoagulant effect. In fact, heparan sulfate proteoglycans, binding to SARS-CoV-2 spike proteins, decrease host protein binding capability and reduce cytokine cascade.[63]

Echocardiography

Regarding instrumental examinations in COVID-19 patients, the use of echocardiogram should be limited in order to limit unnecessary contacts among health care providers and patients.[50] Echocardiography should be performed only if crucial for immediate therapeutic management of critically ill patients.[50] In this case, transthoracic echocardiography must be chosen over transesophageal echocardiography, thereby avoiding the creation of aerosols.[50,64] Transesophageal echocardiography should be avoided for early initiation of anticoagulation in new-onset AF, or maintenance of anticoagulant therapy in patients with known AF.[65] Cardiac computed tomography may be an alternative to transesophageal echocardiography, as it allows ruling out the presence of a left atrial appendage thrombus before cardioversion is performed.[66]

Ablation Procedure

Catheter ablation for AF patients with an ongoing infection is contraindicated; this same criterion applies to COVID-19 patients. Therefore, both AF or AFL ablation procedures should be postponed to optimize antiarrhythmic therapy and control/correct all COVID-19 and non–COVID-19–related modifiable risk factors.[50,67] A different scenario is represented by AF/AFL patients showing evidence of tachycardiomyopathy or syncope; in these patients, an early ablation is pivotal to prevent cardiac remodeling and dysfunction and improve outcomes.[68] Also, ablation of drug-refractory AF and AFL with repeated emergency room visits should be performed within less than 3 months.[50,69–71] Of note, universal testing is of utmost importance to create a safe workplace for patients and health care workers, as asymptomatic carriers can be highly contagious and could be unexpectedly admitted.[72] In case of intubation procedure, this needs to be done out of the electrophysiology laboratory to prevent contamination.

Follow-up in COVID-19 Patients Suffering from Arrhythmias

The follow-up of patients suffering from arrhythmias must be safe in order to prevent patients from being reinfected by COVID-19. Indeed, as the pandemic progressed, telemedicine has been extensively adopted,[73,74] allowing face-to-face outpatient appointments to be replaced by teleconsultations.[75,76] In the TeleCheck-AF project, telemedicine was implemented with remote monitoring of rhythm and frequency of AF, allowing a

Table 1
Interactions between medications for AF and COVID-19

Rate Control Drugs	Remdesivir	Hydroxychloroquine	Azithromycin
β-Blockers			
Atenolol	-	-	-
Bisoprolol	-	-	-
Metoprolol	-	-	-
Propranolol	-	-	-
Nondihydropyridine calcium channel blockers			
Diltiazem	-	-	-
Verapamil	-	↑	-
Others			
Digoxin	-	↑↑	-
Rhythm control drugs			
Amiodarone	-	↑↑↑	↑↑↑
Dronedarone	No data available	↑↑↑	↑↑↑
Flecainide	-	↑↑↑	↑↑
Propafenone	-	-	↑↑↑
Oral anticoagulants			
Apixaban	-	↑	↑↑
Edoxaban	-	↑↑	↑↑↑
Rivaroxaban	-	↑	↑↑
Dabigatran	-	↑↑	↑↑
Warfarin	-	-	-

↑↑↑: Potential substantially increased exposure of the medications; these drugs should not be prescribed together.
↑↑: Potential moderately increased exposure of the medications; dosage adjustment or close monitoring may be required.
↑: Potential mildly increased exposure of the medications; the interactions are weak.
-: No significant effects.

complete management of patients, thanks to a mobile phone app using photoplethysmography technology through the built-in camera.[77] Probably, this model of outpatient management of arrhythmias, thanks to the new wearable technologies, leading to the reduction of the number of hospital visits and health care costs, will remain even after the pandemic and represent an additional weapon in the diagnosis and management of arrhythmias in the near future.[78]

SUMMARY

Cardiac arrhythmias occur in 6% to 17% of COVID-19 patients. Their prevalence is significantly higher (up to 44%) in patients admitted to intensive care unit, becoming the second most frequent complication after acute respiratory distress syndrome. Supraventricular arrhythmias, mainly AF, are more frequent than ventricular ones. Several mechanisms can contribute to an increased risk of cardiac arrhythmias during COVID-19 infection, ranging from direct myocardial damage to electrolyte imbalance. The main aim of COVID-19–related supraventricular arrhythmia management is to establish a safe treatment plan according to each patient's overall clinical conditions, keep in mind any possible drug-to-drug interactions, and minimize the risk of exposure for the staff and other non–COVID-19 patients.

CLINICS CARE POINTS

- Arrhythmogenesis is correlated to several pathophysiological mechanisms: hypoxia, myocardial ischemia, inflammation, electrolyte and fluid imbalance.
- Rate Control should be preferred in critically ill COVID-19 patients.- Atrial fibrillation is an indipendent predictor of mortality.
- COVID-19 patients who experienced atrial fibrillation should be monitored to evaluate the burden of arrhythmia.

DISCLOSURE

Dr J.D. Burkhardt is a consultant for Biosense Webster and Stereotaxis. Dr L. Di Biase is a consultant for Biosense Webster, Boston Scientific, Stereotaxis, and St. Jude Medical; and has received speaker honoraria from Medtronic, Atricure, EPiEP, and Biotronik. Dr A. Natale has received speaker honoraria from Boston Scientific, Biosense Webster, St. Jude Medical, Biotronik, and Medtronic; and is a consultant for Biosense Webster, St. Jude Medical, and Janssen. All other authors have reported that they have no relationships relevant to the contents of this article to disclose.

REFERENCES

1. Lipsitch M, Swerdlow DL, Finelli L. Defining the epidemiology of covid-19 — studies needed. N Engl J Med 2020;382:1194–6.

2. Jee Y. WHO international health regulations emergency committee for the COVID-19 outbreak. Epidemiol Health 2020;42:e2020013.

3. Vetta F. Coronavirus disease 2019 (COVID-19) and cardiovascular disease: a Vicious circle. J Cardiol Cardiovasc Res 2020. https://doi.org/10.37191/Mapsci-JCCR-1(1)-010.

4. Shi S, Qin M, Shen B, et al. Association of cardiac injury with mortality in hospitalized patients with COVID-19 in Wuhan, China. JAMA Cardiol 2020;5:802.

5. Della Rocca DG, Magnocavallo M, Lavalle C, et al. Evidence of systemic endothelial injury and Microthrombosis in hospitalized COVID-19 patients at different Stages of the disease. J Thromb Thrombolysis 2020. https://doi.org/10.1007/s11239-020-02330-1.

6. Lala A, Johnson KW, Januzzi JL, et al. Prevalence and Impact of myocardial injury in patients hospitalized with COVID-19 infection. J Am Coll Cardiol 2020;76:533–46.

7. Cui S, Chen S, Li X, et al. Prevalence of venous thromboembolism in patients with severe novel coronavirus pneumonia. J Thromb Haemost 2020;18:1421–4.

8. Driggin E, Madhavan MV, Bikdeli B, et al. Cardiovascular considerations for patients, health care workers, and health systems during the COVID-19 pandemic. J Am Coll Cardiol 2020;75:2352–71.

9. Wang D, Hu B, Hu C, et al. Clinical characteristics of 138 hospitalized patients with 2019 novel coronavirus–infected pneumonia in Wuhan, China. JAMA 2020;323:1061.

10. Cheng P, Zhu H, Witteles RM, et al. Cardiovascular risks in patients with COVID-19: potential mechanisms and areas of uncertainty. Curr Cardiol Rep 2020;22:34.

11. Dherange P, Lang J, Qian P, et al. Arrhythmias and COVID-19. JACC: Clin Electrophysiol 2020;6:1193–204.

12. Bhatla A, Mayer MM, Adusumalli S, et al. COVID-19 and cardiac arrhythmias. Heart Rhythm 2020;17: 1439–44.

13. Berman JP, Abrams MP, Kushnir A, et al. Cardiac electrophysiology consultative experience at the epicenter of the COVID-19 pandemic in the United States. Indian Pacing Electrophysiol J 2020;20: 250–6.

14. Peltzer B, Manocha KK, Ying X, et al. Outcomes and mortality associated with atrial arrhythmias among patients hospitalized with COVID-19. J Cardiovasc Electrophysiol 2020;31:3077–85.

15. Xiong T-Y, Redwood S, Prendergast B, et al. Coronaviruses and the cardiovascular system: acute and long-term Implications. Eur Heart J 2020;41: 1798–800.

16. Lazzerini PE, Boutjdir M, Capecchi PL. COVID-19, arrhythmic risk, and inflammation: mind the gap. Circulation 2020;142:7–9.

17. Kolettis TM. Coronary artery disease and ventricular Tachyarrhythmia: pathophysiology and treatment. Curr Opin Pharmacol 2013;13:210–7.

18. Hu H, Ma F, Wei X, et al. Coronavirus Fulminant myocarditis treated with glucocorticoid and human Immunoglobulin. Eur Heart J 2021;42:206.

19. Denham NC, Pearman CM, Caldwell JL, et al. Calcium in the pathophysiology of atrial fibrillation and heart failure. Front Physiol 2018;9:1380.

20. Lindner D, Fitzek A, Bräuninger H, et al. Association of cardiac infection with SARS-CoV-2 in confirmed COVID-19 autopsy cases. JAMA Cardiol 2020;5:1281.

21. Siripanthong B, Nazarian S, Muser D, et al. Recognizing COVID-19–related myocarditis: the possible pathophysiology and proposed guideline for diagnosis and management. Heart Rhythm 2020;17: 1463–71.

22. Wrapp D, Wang N, Corbett KS, et al. Cryo-EM structure of the 2019-NCoV spike in the prefusion conformation. Science 2020;367:1260–3.

23. South AM, Diz DI, Chappell MC. COVID-19, ACE2, and the cardiovascular consequences. Am J Physiol Heart Circ Physiol 2020;318:H1084–90.

24. Oudit GY, Kassiri Z, Jiang C, et al. SARS-coronavirus Modulation of myocardial ACE2 expression and inflammation in patients with SARS. Eur J Clin Invest 2009;39:618–25.

25. Tse G, Yeo JM, Chan YW, et al. What is the arrhythmic Substrate in viral myocarditis? Insights from clinical and animal studies. Front Physiol 2016;7:308.

26. Huertas A, Montani D, Savale L, et al. Endothelial cell dysfunction: a major player in SARS-CoV-2 infection (COVID-19)? Eur Respir J 2020;56: 2001634.

27. Madjid M, Vela D, Khalili-Tabrizi H, et al. Systemic infections cause exaggerated local inflammation in atherosclerotic coronary arteries: clues to the

triggering effect of acute infections on acute coronary syndromes. Tex Heart Inst J 2007;34:11–8.

28. Della Rocca DG, Pepine CJ. Endothelium as a predictor of adverse outcomes: endothelium as a predictor of adverse outcomes. Clin Cardiol 2010;33: 730–2.

29. Musher DM, Abers MS, Corrales-Medina VF. Acute infection and myocardial Infarction. N Engl J Med 2019;380:171–6.

30. Della Rocca DG, Pepine CJ. Some Thoughts on the continuing dilemma of angina pectoris. Eur Heart J 2014;35:1361–4.

31. Pober JS, Sessa WC. Evolving Functions of endothelial cells in inflammation. Nat Rev Immunol 2007;7:803–15.

32. Varga Z, Flammer AJ, Steiger P, et al. Endothelial cell infection and endotheliitis in COVID-19. Lancet 2020;395:1417–8.

33. Huang C, Wang Y, Li X, et al. Clinical features of patients infected with 2019 novel coronavirus in Wuhan, China. Lancet 2020;395:497–506.

34. Lee S-H, Chen Y-C, Chen Y-J, et al. Tumor Necrosis factor-α alters calcium handling and increases arrhythmogenesis of pulmonary vein cardiomyocytes. Life Sci 2007;80:1806–15.

35. Aschar-Sobbi R, Izaddoustdar F, Korogyi AS, et al. Increased atrial arrhythmia Susceptibility induced by Intense endurance exercise in Mice requires TNFα. Nat Commun 2015;6:6018.

36. Mohanty S, Trivedi C, Della Rocca DG, et al. Thromboembolic risk in atrial fibrillation patients with left atrial scar post-extensive ablation. JACC: Clin Electrophysiol 2021;7:308–18.

37. Lazzerini PE, Laghi-Pasini F, Acampa M, et al. Systemic inflammation Rapidly induces Reversible atrial electrical remodeling: the role of interleukin-6–mediated changes in connexin expression. JAHA 2019;8. https://doi.org/10.1161/JAHA.118.011006.

38. Canpolat U, Mohanty S, Trivedi C, et al. Association of Fragmented QRS with left atrial Scarring in patients with persistent atrial fibrillation undergoing Radiofrequency catheter ablation. Heart Rhythm 2020; 17:203–10.

39. Puntmann VO, Taylor PC, Barr A, et al. Towards understanding the phenotypes of myocardial involvement in the presence of Self-limiting and Sustained systemic inflammation: a Magnetic Resonance Imaging study. Rheumatology 2010;49:528–35.

40. El-Sherif N, Turitto G. Electrolyte disorders and arrhythmogenesis. Cardiol J 2011;18:233–45.

41. Chen D, Li X, Song Q, et al. Assessment of hypokalemia and clinical characteristics in patients with coronavirus disease 2019 in Wenzhou, China. JAMA Netw Open 2020;3:e2011122.

42. Diao B, Wang C, Wang R, et al. Human Kidney is a Target for novel severe acute respiratory syndrome coronavirus 2 infection. Nat Commun 2021;12:2506.

43. Krijthe BP, Heeringa J, Kors JA, et al. Serum potassium levels and the risk of atrial fibrillation. Int J Cardiol 2013;168:5411–5.

44. Desai AD, Boursiquot BC, Melki L, et al. Management of arrhythmias associated with COVID-19. Curr Cardiol Rep 2021;23:2.

45. Chen Q, Xu J, Gianni C, et al. Simple electrocardiographic criteria for Rapid Identification of Wide QRS complex Tachycardia: the new limb lead algorithm. Heart Rhythm 2020;17:431–8.

46. Coromilas EJ, Kochav S, Goldenthal I, et al. Worldwide survey of COVID-19–associated arrhythmias. Circ Arrhythmia Electrophysiol 2021;14. https://doi.org/10.1161/CIRCEP.120.009458.

47. Goyal P, Choi JJ, Pinheiro LC, et al. Clinical characteristics of covid-19 in New York city. N Engl J Med 2020;382:2372–4.

48. Garcia-Zamora S, Lee S, Haseeb S, et al. Arrhythmias and electrocardiographic findings in coronavirus disease 2019: a Systematic review and meta-analysis. Pacing Clin Electrophysiol 2021;44:1062–74.

49. Zareini B, Rajan D, El-Sheikh M, et al. Cardiac arrhythmias in patients hospitalized with COVID-19: the ACOVID study. Heart Rhythm O2 2021;2:304–8.

50. The European Society for Cardiology. ESC Guidance for the Diagnosis and Management of CV Disease during the COVID-19 Pandemic. Available at: https://www.escardio.org/Education/COVID-19-and-Cardiology.

51. Saenz LC, Miranda A, Speranza R, et al. Recommendations for the organization of electrophysiology and cardiac pacing Services during the COVID-19 pandemic: Latin American heart rhythm Society (LAHRS) in collaboration with: Colombian college of electrophysiology, argentinian Society of cardiac electrophysiology (SADEC), Brazilian Society of cardiac arrhythmias (SOBRAC), Mexican Society of cardiac electrophysiology (SOMEEC). J Interv Card Electrophysiol 2020;59:307–13.

52. Goldschlager N, Epstein AE, Naccarelli GV, et al. A practical guide for clinicians who treat patients with amiodarone: 2007. Heart Rhythm 2007;4: 1250–9.

53. Russo V, Carbone A, Mottola FF, et al. Effect of Triple combination therapy with lopinavir-ritonavir, azithromycin, and hydroxychloroquine on QT Interval and arrhythmic risk in hospitalized COVID-19 patients. Front Pharmacol 2020;11:582348.

54. Lavalle C, Trivigno S, Vetta G, et al. Flecainide in ventricular arrhythmias: from old Myths to new perspectives. JCM 2021;10:3696.

55. Ganatra S, Dani SS, Shah S, et al. Management of cardiovascular disease during coronavirus disease (COVID-19) pandemic. Trends Cardiovasc Med 2020;30:315–25.

56. Capel RA, Herring N, Kalla M, et al. Hydroxychloroquine reduces heart rate by Modulating the

hyperpolarization-activated current if: novel electro-physiological Insights and therapeutic potential. Heart Rhythm 2015;12:2186–94.

57. Hindricks G, Potpara T, Dagres N, et al. 2020 ESC guidelines for the diagnosis and management of atrial fibrillation developed in collaboration with the European association for cardio-Thoracic Surgery (EACTS). Eur Heart J 2021;42:373–498.

58. Agarwal S, Agarwal SK. Lopinavir-Ritonavir in SARS-CoV-2 infection and drug-drug interactions with cardioactive medications. Cardiovasc Drugs Ther 2021;35:427–40.

59. Testa S, Prandoni P, Paoletti O, et al. Direct oral anti-coagulant plasma levels' Striking increase in severe COVID-19 respiratory syndrome patients treated with antiviral agents: the cremona experience. J Thromb Haemost 2020;18:1320–3.

60. Gawałko M, Kapłon-Cieślicka A, Hohl M, et al. COVID-19 associated atrial fibrillation: Incidence, putative mechanisms and potential clinical Implications. IJC Heart & Vasculature 2020;30:100631.

61. Lavalle C, Di Lullo L, Bellasi A, et al. Adverse drug Reactions during Real-life use of direct oral anticoagulants in Italy: an update Based on data from the Italian national pharmacovigilance network. Cardiorenal Med 2020;10:266–76.

62. Holbrook A, Schulman S, Witt DM, et al. Evidence-based management of anticoagulant therapy: antithrombotic therapy and prevention of thrombosis, 9th ed: American college of chest physicians evidence-Based clinical practice guidelines. Chest 2012;141:e152S–84S.

63. Yu M, Zhang T, Zhang W, et al. Elucidating the interactions between heparin/heparan Sulfate and SARS-CoV-2-related proteins—an important strategy for developing novel therapeutics for the COVID-19 pandemic. Front Mol Biosci 2021;7:628551.

64. Irons JF, Pavey W, Bennetts JS, et al. COVID-19 safety: aerosol-generating procedures and cardiothoracic Surgery and anaesthesia - Australian and New Zealand consensus Statement. Med J Aust 2021;214:40–4.

65. Gedikli Ö, Mohanty S, Trivedi C, et al. Impact of dense "Smoke" detected on Transesophageal echocardiography on stroke risk in patients with atrial fibrillation undergoing catheter ablation. Heart Rhythm 2019;16:351–7.

66. Pathan F, Hecht H, Narula J, et al. Roles of Transesophageal echocardiography and cardiac computed tomography for evaluation of left atrial thrombus and associated pathology: a review and critical analysis. JACC Cardiovasc Imaging 2018;11:616–27.

67. Calkins H, Hindricks G, Cappato R, et al. 2017 HRS/EHRA/ECAS/APHRS/SOLAECE expert consensus Statement on catheter and Surgical ablation of atrial fibrillation. Europace 2018;20:e1–160.

68. Della Rocca DG, Santini L, Forleo GB, et al. Novel perspectives on arrhythmia-Induced cardiomyopathy: pathophysiology, clinical manifestations and an update on invasive management Strategies. Cardiol Rev 2015;23:135–41.

69. Della Rocca DG, Mohanty S, Mohanty P, et al. Long-term outcomes of catheter ablation in patients with longstanding persistent atrial fibrillation lasting less than 2 Years. J Cardiovasc Electrophysiol 2018;29:1607–15.

70. Della Rocca DG, Di Biase L, Mohanty S, et al. Targeting non-pulmonary vein triggers in persistent atrial fibrillation: results from a prospective, Multicentre, observational Registry. EP Europace 2021. https://doi.org/10.1093/europace/euab161. euab161.

71. Della Rocca DG, Tarantino N, Trivedi C, et al. Non-pulmonary vein triggers in nonparoxysmal atrial fibrillation: Implications of pathophysiology for catheter ablation. J Cardiovasc Electrophysiol 2020;31:2154–67.

72. Mohanty S, Lakkireddy D, Trivedi C, et al. Creating a safe workplace by universal testing of SARS-CoV-2 infection in asymptomatic patients and healthcare workers in the electrophysiology units: a Multicenter experience. J Interv Card Electrophysiol 2020. https://doi.org/10.1007/s10840-020-00886-9.

73. Forleo GB, Tesauro M, Panattoni G, et al. Impact of continuous Intracardiac ST-Segment monitoring on Mid-term outcomes of ICD-Implanted patients with coronary artery disease. Early results of a prospective comparison with conventional ICD outcomes. Heart 2012;98:402–7.

74. Della Rocca DG, Albanese M, Placidi F, et al. Feasibility of automated detection of Sleep apnea using Implantable pacemakers and defibrillators: a comparison with Simultaneous polysomnography Recording. J Interv Card Electrophysiol 2019;56:327–33.

75. Piro A, Magnocavallo M, Della Rocca DG, et al. Management of cardiac Implantable electronic device follow-up in COVID-19 pandemic: lessons learned during Italian lockdown. J Cardiovasc Electrophysiol 2020;31:2814–23.

76. Magnocavallo M, Bernardini A, Mariani MV, et al. Home delivery of the communicator for remote monitoring of cardiac Implantable devices: a Multicenter experience during the covid-19 lockdown. Pacing Clin Electrophysiol 2021;44:995–1003.

77. Gawałko M, Duncker D, Manninger M, et al. The European TeleCheck-AF project on remote app-Based management of atrial fibrillation during the COVID-19 pandemic: centre and patient experiences. Europace 2021;23:1003–15.

78. Caillol T, Strik M, Ramirez FD, et al. Accuracy of a Smartwatch-derived ECG for diagnosing Bradyarrhythmias, Tachyarrhythmias, and cardiac ischemia. Circ Arrhythmia Electrophysiol 2021;14.

Prevalence, Outcomes, and Management of Ventricular Arrhythmias in COVID-19 Patients

Nicola Tarantino, MD[a], Domenico G. Della Rocca, MD[b], Fengwei Zou, MD[a], Aung Lin, MD[a], Andrea Natale, MD[b,c,d], Luigi Di Biase, MD, PhD[a,b],*

KEYWORDS

- Arrhythmias • COVID-19 • Complications • Management • Outcomes • SARS-CoV-2
- Ventricular tachycardia

KEY POINTS

- Ventricular arrhythmias (VAs) affect a modest proportion of patients with SARS-CoV-2, sometimes representing the only initial symptom.
- The cause of VAs in the setting of acute COVID-19 infection is multifactorial because of direct and indirect myocardial involvement.
- Admission to ICU, use of pressors, pre-existing cardiac disease, but neither QT interval nor left ventricular ejection fraction are consistently associated with such complication.
- Sustained VAs correlate with increased mortality, albeit most of the cardiac arrests originate from not-shockable rhythms.
- Treatment options include correction of metabolic disorder, discontinuation of QT-prolonging agents, antiarrhythmics (especially amiodarone), and ablation in case of a ventricular storm.

INTRODUCTION

At the time of writing the present article, SARS-CoV-2, aka COVID-19, has reportedly hit almost 180 million people globally in less than 18 months since its official identification and disclosure as pandemic.[1] Initially announced as a severe acute respiratory syndrome due to a novel strain of coronavirus, after the acronym SARS-CoV-2, the first pandemic of the third millennium was unexpectedly far from being an isolated respiratory condition. Instead, a multitude of signs and symptoms, sometimes representing the only atypical manifestation of the disease, have been described with alacrity, making the COVID-19 indeed configuring as a systemic disease requiring a multidisciplinary care.

Pertaining to the cardiovascular complications or manifestations of the SARS-CoV-2, in the present article, we offer an overview of the ventricular arrhythmias related to acute COVID-19 infections, discussing the prevalence, the possible mechanisms due to direct or indirect virus involvement, and the currently proposed therapeutic options.

Funding: None declared.
[a] Montefiore Medical Center, 111 E 210th street, Bronx, NY 10467, USA; [b] Texas Cardiac Arrhythmia Institute at St. David's Medical Center, 3000 N I-35, Suite 720, Austin, TX 78705, USA; [c] Scripps Interventional Car, 9834 Genesee Ave, La Jolla, CA 92037, USA; [d] Health Education Campus, 9501 Euclid Ave, Cleveland, OH 44106, USA
* Corresponding author. Montefiore Medical Center, 111 E 210th street, Bronx, NY 10467, USA
E-mail address: dibbia@gmail.com

Card Electrophysiol Clin 14 (2022) 11–20
https://doi.org/10.1016/j.ccep.2021.10.002
1877-9182/22/© 2021 Elsevier Inc. All rights reserved.

EPIDEMIOLOGY AND CLINICAL OUTCOMES
Prevalence and Nature of VAs

Mitacchione and colleagues described the first case of ventricular storm (12 episodes of sustained ventricular tachycardias [VTs]) with concomitant COVID-19 infection in a patient with defibrillator (ICD) and ischemic cardiomyopathy (ejection fraction = 34%) admitted to an Italian hospital for respiratory distress.[2] ICD interrogation showed sustained and nonsustained monomorphic VTs since days before the admission. The authors excluded iatrogenic causes because the systemic use of QT-prolonging immunomodulators and antimicrobials was not recommended at that time, and the VT was probably due to other mechanisms (see paragraph 4). This insightful report suggests that VAs could be the first sign of latent infection in susceptible patients with structural heart disease.

In addition, two descriptions of polymorphic ventricular tachycardia (PMVT) in the settings of prolonged and normal QT, respectively, were also reported.[3,4] Of interest, two separate cases of newly diagnosed Brugada syndrome were reported, one presenting as an asymptomatic coved-type pattern during febrile peak,[5] and the other as PMVT due to fever and drug-induced bradycardia.[6]

The overall prevalence of VAs in COVID-19 patients ranges between 0.15% and 8% (**Table 1**).[7,8] Such a discrepancy stems from the definition of VAs and subpopulations analyzed. The first series by Guo showed that malignant arrhythmias were relatively more common in patients with cardiac injury—defined as troponin T elevation—(11% vs 5% over a total of 187 individuals).[8] A retrospective study of 700 patients differentiated the prevalence between patients admitted to intensive care unit (ICU) compared with nonintensive care settings.[7] In total, only one patient had a life-threatening torsade de pointes (TdP) in ICU (1.4% vs none in the comparison group). Similarly, nonsustained episodes were more common in critical patients (8% vs 0.6%). In line with this analysis, a Scandinavian group observed that incidence of VAs in ICU patients was about 3% (n = 2/155),[9] yet, according to a larger cohort of 1053 hospitalized patients, nonsustained episodes are far less prevalent than malignant VAs (0.7% vs ≈ 3%).[10]

Lastly, no data are currently available in regard to VAs incidence in COVID-19 patients with implanted cardiac devices treated conservatively at home. In this regard, it is worth carrying out such analysis, as experienced in different settings.[11]

Clinical Value and Outcomes

Despite the slight numerical divergence, it is worth noting that the occurrence of VAs consistently clustered with complicated hospitalizations, suggesting that ventricular arrhythmias are a marker of severe systemic disease.[7,10] Indeed, besides anecdotic cases of VA survivors,[2–4,6] the mortality at 1 month is substantially higher in patients experiencing arrhythmias of ventricular nature (VT or ventricular fibrillation [VF], 59% vs 16% in controls; $P<.001$, respectively).[10] On the contrary, nonsustained episodes of VAs do not seem to predict mortality within a year.[7]

Furthermore, another detailed breakdown of the relationship between VAs and clinical outcomes argues against the role of malignant VTs as the primary/initial cause of death. For instance, as reported by two different groups, a nonshockable rhythm was the predominant cause of cardiac arrest/death (90% in both studies).[7,10] Correspondingly, in a series of 140 patients admitted on telemetry monitor, fatal VAs were noted in only 12% of deceased patients (6/52).[12] All the events were represented by VF, 1 patient survived, and 2 autopsy examinations suggested that the initial cause of death was pulmonary rather than cardiac.

The prevalence and clinical significance of premature ventricular contractions (PVCs) in the setting of acute infection were less investigated; although subjects with SARS-CoV-2 infection can initially complain of palpitations (7%),[13] dedicated analysis is scarce. An Italian study showed that 4% (n = 13/324) of COVID-19 positive subjects admitted to the emergency department presented ventricular ectopy,[14] compared to 13% of 1053 hospitalized patients (n = 137).[10] Despite the evidence that PVCs are seen in cases of novel coronavirus-related myocarditis,[15,16] the positive predictive value for cardiac involvement is poor,[17] and likewise the association with mortality is borderline (HR = 2.79; 95% CI, 1.00–7.79; $P = .051$).[14]

MECHANISMS AND PREDICTORS OF VAs IN THE SETTING OF ACUTE COVID-19 INFECTION

A broad number of articles discuss the possible causes of VAs during acute COVID-19. For the sake of simplification, herein we distinguish between intrinsic and extrinsic causes, depending on the direct or indirect role of the pathogenic agent. The formers can be divided into 2 types: primary intrinsic (directly due to the interaction between the virus and the cardiomyocyte) and secondary intrinsic (after the immune response to the systemic infection; **Fig. 1**). Overall, rarely a

Table 1
Synopsis of the studies reporting the prevalence of VAs in the setting of acute COVID-19 infection

Author and Date	Sample	Number and Type of VA	QT/QT-Prolonging Agents	Underlying Cardiac Disease	Primary Cause Hypothesized	Management	Outcome
Mitacchione et al,[2] 2020	1	VT storm	• NS • none	ICM	• Systemic inflammation • Pre-existing cardiac disease	VT ablation with remote navigation control	Discharged
Elsad et al,[3] 2020	1	Bradycardia-induced TdP; VF	• 650 ms • none	None	Multiorgan failure	Lidocaine Magnesium Dopamine Transcutaneous pacing	Discharged
O'Brien et al,[4] 2020	1	PMVT	• 460 ms • Hydroxymorphone • Amiodarone[a] • Trazodone	None	Multiorgan failure	Discontinuation of amiodarone Lidocaine Metoprolol	Demise
Chang et al,[5] 2020	1	NS	NS	Brugada	• Systemic inflammation • Fever • Congenital channelopathy	Observation	Discharged
Tsimpoulis et al,[6] 2020	1	PMVT	• 422 ms • HCQ • AZT • Propofol • Dexmedetomidine	Brugada	• Systemic inflammation • Fever • Congenital channelopathy • Pressors	Supportive care	Demise
Bathla et al,[7] 2020	700	• 1 TdP • 10 NSVT	• NS • NS	• De novo left ventricular dysfunction • NS	• Multiorgan failure	NS	• 10 survived • 1 demise
Guo et al,[8] 2020	187	11 VT/VF	• NS • NS	NS	• Systemic inflammation • Cardiac injury	NS	NS

(continued on next page)

Table 1
(continued)

Author and Date	Sample	Number and Type of VA	QT/QT-Prolonging Agents	Underlying Cardiac Disease	Primary Cause Hypothesized	Management	Outcome
Wetterslev et al,[9] 2021	155	2 NS	• NS • NS	NS	• Multiorgan failure • Pressors	NS	NS
Peltzer et al,[10] 2020	1053	• 137 PVC • 7 NSVT • 13 VT • 9 PMVT • 8 VF	• NS/ 4 of the 745 using HCQ+ had PMVT	NS	• Multiorgan failure • Pressors	NS	59% of patients with VA died
Turagam et al,[11] 2020	140	• 6 VF • 1 VT	• NS • 107/140 used HCQ; - 62/140 used HCQ + AZT	NS	• Multiorgan failure/ pressors (5/7) • NS in one VF patient • Pre-existing cardiac disease (VT patient)	NS	• 6 demises (VF group) • 1 survived (VT patient)
Mesquita D,[12] 2021	692	2 VT	Prolonged in both	NS	• Multiorgan failure • QT prolongation • Pre-existing cardiac condition	NS	Demise in both[b]
Lanza et al,[14] 2021	324	13 PVC	• NS • NS	NS	NS	NS	4 demises
Perretto et al,[15] 2021	7	• 2 PVC/NSVT • 1 VT • 1 VF	• Normal; • HCQ/AZT in 3/4 pts with VAs	CAD	• Myocarditis • Pre-existing cardiac disease • Pressors	• Amiodarone in 1 pt with NSVT • Metoprolol/ Bisoprolol in the others	Discharged (ICD in pt with VF and in 1 with NSVT). All alive at 6 months
D'Ascenzo et al,[30] 2021	779	38 VT/VF	• NS • NS	CAD	ACS Multifactorial	NS	NS

Saleh M,[39] 2020	201	• 7 NSVT • 1 VT	• NS • All pts were treated with HCQ, 119 with also AZT	No	• Myocarditis in pt with VT • Hypoxemia and systemic inflammation in the others	NS	• 6 discharged • 2 demises (1 with VT)
Gasparetti A,[40] 2020	649	• 3 VF • 4 VT	• NS • All pts were treated with HCQ	6 ICM	• ACS in pts with VF • Multiorgan failure in the remainder	• HCQ discontinuation	3 demises (VF group)

Abbreviations: ACS, acute coronary syndrome; AZT, azithromycin; CAD, coronary artery disease; HCQ, hydroxychloroquine; ICM, ischemic cardiomyopathy; NS, nonspecified; NSVT, nonsustained VT; PMVT, polymorphic ventricular tachycardia; pts, patients; PVC, premature ventricular contraction; TdP, torsade de pointes; VF, ventricular fibrillation; VT, ventricular tachycardia.

[a] For atrial fibrillation with rapid ventricular response.

[b] Due to respiratory failure.

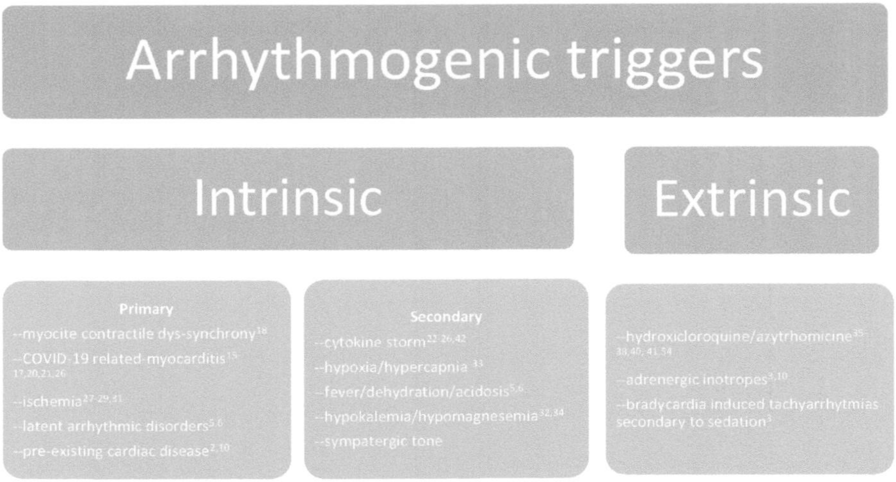

Fig. 1. Schematic classification of VA causes in COVID-19 patients.

single factor can be pointed as the source of VA; instead, plural elements could affect the electrical vulnerability of the ventricles.[18]

Intrinsic Factors

A brilliant in vitro model showed that infected cardiomyocytes derived from a human pluripotent staminal cell exhibit a significant reduction of the contractile activity measured as beats per minute (4 vs 9 in controls) and a greater extent of contraction dis-synchrony compared with mock SARS-CoV-2 negative cultures.[19] Such effect became even more prominent after 48 hours of treatment with interleukin-6. In fact, even though the presence of the virus in cardiac tissue or evidence of myocarditis have been inconsistently detected,[20–22] cytokines surge from the systemic immune response are alone sufficient to dysregulate calcium handling, modulate ion channels expression, increase fibrosis, and exert a negative inotropic effect, ultimately enhancing the susceptibility to VAs.[23–27] For example, late VAs and epicardial fibrosis at the magnetic resonance were documented in one case months after the resolution of the acute illness.[28]

COVID-19 can provoke cardiac ischemia as well, due to both hypoxia/demanding mechanism,[29] but also as it can eminently be thrombogenic and cause coronary microemboli and acute coronary syndromes (ACSs).[30,31] The relationship with sustained VAs, however, does not differ from negative controls admitted with ACSs (4.9% vs 6.8%, P = ns).[32] Beyond the direct involvement of the heart, systemic metabolic derangements such as acidosis, hypercapnia, hypokalemia, dehydration, and catecholamines surge do precipitate VAs.[33–37] Also, fever can

incidentally unmask Brugada pattern in predisposed subjects,[5,6] and obviously, patients with pre-existing cardiomyopathy are more prone to develop VAs in the setting of SARS-CoV-2 infection.[2,10]

Extrinsic Factors and Predictors of VAs

VAs can also be iatrogenic. Based on the evidence that hydroxychloroquine and chloroquine inhibit lysosome turnover, and consequently the antigen presentation initiating the immune response,[38] there has been a large empirical use of antimalarial drugs at the beginning of the pandemic with the purpose to damper the adverse events and the hospitalization duration. However, the most concerning side effects of hydroxychloroquine are QT prolongation and TdP, especially if combined with antimicrobial prophylaxis with azithromycin or lopinavir/ritonavir.[39,40] Indeed, the duration of phase 2 of the action potential is prolonged through hydroxychloroquine inhibition of the hERG channels, slowing the potassium rapid inward currents (iKr), and by means of sodium current enhancement exerted by azithromycin on SC5NA.[41–43] Repolarization prolongation by 10 to 50 ms is relatively frequent (5%–50%),[10,34,35,44] and in one series of 201 patients treated with empirical prophylaxis, 18 (11%) developed QTc prolongation greater than 500 ms, albeit only one patient had sustained VT (0.5%), and no TdP was recorded.[34] In another series, no difference in VAs incidence was seen between patients treated with antimalarial agents versus controls,[10] whereas Gasparetti and colleagues concluded that the 3 VF observed in 28 patients admitted in ICU (10%) were due to ongoing ACS and not hydroxychloroquine-induced QT.[37]

Therefore, QT prolongation inconsistently predicts VAs in COVID-19 patients,[3,10,35] likewise hydroxychloroquine is rarely associated with malignant arrhythmias (<1%).[10,35,37] ST-T wave changes seemingly are not related to VAs[45]; however, elevated markers of cardiac injury (troponin, natriuretic peptide) and systemic inflammation (ie, C-reactive protein, interleukin-6) are significantly higher in patients presenting life-threatening arrhythmias,[3,8,9,46,47] nonetheless it is not univocally acknowledged.[10] Differently, a high dose of pressors seems to correlate with VAs incidence, both due to adrenergic stimulation and also for an implication of severe cardiogenic shock, whereas the value of admission left ventricular function is controversial.[8–11,15,43]

THERAPEUTIC OPTIONS

If supportive management, including correction of electrolyte and acid/base derangement, fluid repletion, blood transfusion, coronary or pulmonary reperfusion, is not adequate, rationale antiarrhythmic strategies should be adopted. Sedatives and anesthetics should be titrated down or discontinued when identified as the cause of bradycardia or QT prolongation,[4] and standard dose of beta blockers is certainly useful compatibly with the cardiac output.

Thirty-four percent of the 447 respondents (n = 150) to a global survey (March-April 2020) admitted to using amiodarone for VAs treatment, whereas 15% (n = 64) disclosed having used lidocaine or mexiletine for the same purpose. Other class III agents (sotalol and dofetilide) were rarely reported.[48] Pulmonary and hepatic toxicity probably refrained most physicians from adopting amiodarone in secondary prevention in patients with a concomitant viral respiratory syndrome often complicated by liver dysfunction.[49]

According to some authors, lung toxicity is more likely to occur in ICU patients in which the oxidative damage of high oxygen partial pressure potentiates the free radicals derived from the iodine accumulated in the alveoli.[50] However, it is worth highlighting that acute lung toxicity is an adverse event reported anecdotally[51,52]; rather, a cumulative dose of 150 g, equivalent to 400 mg daily for 3 months, or 200 mg for more than 18 months are associated with pulmonary injury.[53–56]

On the contrary, liver toxicity requires as high as 300 g of cumulative dose,[57] but according to some German scholars, one-third of the SARS-CoV-2 patients admitted in ICU has shock liver, which may compromise amiodarone metabolism.[45]

In our opinion, the vast experience in daily practice and the existing literature in non-COVID scenarios is more than sufficient to state that amiodarone is efficacious for malignant arrhythmias in COVID-19 patients. Despite isolated warning reports about lung and hepatic toxicity in some subjects with new coronavirus infection,[58–60] the legitimate concern should be the risk of liver injury and of QT prolongation secondary to drug-drug interaction with antimicrobials[36,40]; thus, we think that amiodarone should be cautiously dosed in patients with extreme transaminitis, but still be preferred to other more torsadogenic class III agents. Furthermore, in the case of long QT (>550 ms), the treatment should switch to Ib agents, which can shorten the repolarization.[61]

Interestingly, amiodarone exhibits pleiotropic effects that can interfere with SARS-CoV-2 infection, by altering the ion channels of the endosomal vesicles.[62] Also, it prevents cytokines production supposedly through the same mechanism in lymphocytes in vivo,[63] and additionally presents scavenging effects of oxygen free radicals in vitro.[64] In light of such anti-inflammatory antioxidant properties, amiodarone has been proposed for the treatment of symptomatic patients; besides a single case report,[65] a randomized trial in comparison with verapamil is currently on recruiting (ReCOVery-SIRIO, ClinicalTrials.gov identifier: NCT04351763).[66,67]

ICDs and endocardial ablation should be recommended in agreement with the international guidelines,[68–70] and when available, a remote navigation system should be used for the ablation to minimize the exposure of the medical staff.[2]

SUMMARY

SARS-CoV-2 is a systemic disease that can also impair the electrical stability of the ventricles. Although a direct cardiac infection by the virus is plausible, the host's systemic neuroinflammatory response in addition to metabolic disorders are the main triggers of VAs. The physician should be aware that subjects with pre-existing cardiac disease, admitted to ICU, requiring pressor support are more at risk of developing malignant arrhythmias. Therefore, strict monitoring of drugs interactions and precipitating factors (such as hypoxemia, hypokalemia, acidosis) is essential for primary prevention. Amiodarone is generally safe for the secondary prophylaxis of sustained events, and also might show unexplored antiviral/anti-inflammatory effects in human. Intravenous procainamide, lidocaine, or oral mexiletine are alternatives, albeit the evidence is limited. Contrarily, sotalol and dofetilide should be discouraged, because the more significant torsadogenic effect can be detrimental in such a delicate scenario. Lastly, substrate ablation is recommended in case of refractory episodes, possibly by using a remote navigation system to minimize the contact with the providers.

CLINICS CARE POINTS

- Ventricular arrhythmias prevail in less than 10% (<1–8%) of the patients with acute COVID-19 infection, including premature ventricular contractions and life-threatening events.

- The cause is multifactorial and includes direct virus interaction with cardiomyocytes, the effect of interleukins, neurohormonal output, pre-existing cardiac disease, metabolic disorders, iatrogenic toxicity, and latent congenital arrhythmic disorders precipitated by the systemic illness.

- Although VAs are associated with increased mortality, it does not imply that they are the primary cause of death. In contrast, they express the terminal event of a severe systemic metabolic and inflammatory catastrophe.

- In absence of reversible causes (ie, QT-prolonging agents, hypoxemia, hypokalemia), amiodarone is generally safe if other parameters are monitored (ie, liver function) and could theoretically exhibit pleiotropic beneficial effects on the infection itself. Class I agents represent valid alternatives, and ablation should be performed following the international guidelines, possibly with the help of a robotic navigation system to maximize contact isolation.

DISCLOSURE

Dr A. Natale has received speaker honoraria from Boston Scientific, Biosense Webster, St. Jude Medical, Biotronik, and Medtronic; and is a consultant for Biosense Webster, St. Jude Medical, and Janssen. Dr L. Di Biase is a consultant for Biosense Webster, RMG, Stereotaxis, Boston Scientific, and Abbott. Dr L. Di Biase received speaker honoraria/travel from Medtronic, Atricure, and Biotronik. All other authors have reported that they have no relationships relevant to the contents of this article to disclose.

REFERENCES

1. Available at: https://coronavirus.jhu.edu/map.html. Accessed on June 12, 2021.

2. Mitacchione G, Schiavone M, Gasperetti A, et al. Ventricular tachycardia storm management in a COVID-19 patient: a case report. Eur Heart J Case Rep 2020;4(FI1):1–6.

3. Elsaid O, McCullough PA, Tecson KM, et al. Ventricular fibrillation storm in coronavirus 2019. Am J Cardiol 2020;135:177–80.

4. O'Brien C, Ning N, McAvoy J, et al. Electrical storm in COVID-19. JACC Case Rep 2020;2(9):1256–60.

5. Chang D, Saleh M, Garcia-Bengo Y, et al. COVID-19 infection unmasking brugada syndrome. Heartrhythm Case Rep 2020;6:237–40.

6. Tsimploulis A, Rashba EJ, Rahman T, et al. Fan R Medication unmasked Brugada syndrome and cardiac arrest in a COVID-19 patient. Heartrhythm Case Rep 2020;6(9):554–7.

7. Bhatla A, Mayer MM, Adusumalli S, et al. COVID-19 and cardiac arrhythmias. Heart Rhythm 2020;17(9):1439–44.

8. Guo T, Fan Y, Chen M, et al. Cardiovascular implications of fatal outcomes of patients with coronavirus disease 2019 (COVID-19). JAMA Cardiol 2020;5(7):811–8.

9. Wetterslev M, Jacobsen PK, Hassager C, et al. Cardiac arrhythmias in critically ill patients with coronavirus disease 2019: a retrospective population-based cohort study. Acta Anaesthesiol Scand 2021;65(6):770–7.

10. Peltzer B, Manocha KK, Ying X, et al. Arrhythmic complications of patients hospitalized with COVID-19: incidence, risk factors, and outcomes. Circ Arrhythm Electrophysiol 2020;13(10):e009121.

11. Piro A, Magnocavallo M, Della Rocca DG, et al. Management of cardiac implantable electronic device follow-up in COVID-19 pandemic: Lessons learned during Italian lockdown. J Cardiovasc Electrophysiol 2020;31(11):2814–23.

12. Turagam MK, Musikantow D, Goldman ME, et al. Malignant arrhythmias in patients with COVID-19: incidence, mechanisms, and outcomes. Circ Arrhythm Electrophysiol 2020;13(11):e008920.

13. Liu K, Fang YY, Deng Y, et al. Clinical characteristics of novel coronavirus cases in tertiary hospitals in Hubei Province. Chin Med J (Engl) 2020;133(9):1025–31.

14. Lanza GA, De Vita A, Ravenna SE, et al. Electrocardiographic findings at presentation and clinical outcome in patients with SARS-CoV-2 infection. Europace 2021;23(1):123–9.

15. Peretto G, Villatore A, Rizzo S, et al. The spectrum of COVID-19-associated myocarditis: a patient-tailored multidisciplinary approach. J Clin Med 2021;10(9):1974.

16. Ho JS, Sia CH, Chan MY, et al. Coronavirus-induced myocarditis: a meta-summary of cases. Heart Lung 2020;49(6):681–5.

17. Siripanthong B, Nazarian S, Muser D, et al. Recognizing COVID-19-related myocarditis: the possible

pathophysiology and proposed guideline for diagnosis and management. Heart Rhythm 2020;17(9):1463–71.

18. Della Rocca DG, Santini L, Forleo GB, et al. Novel perspectives on arrhythmia-induced cardiomyopathy: pathophysiology, clinical manifestations and an update on invasive management strategies. Cardiol Rev 2015;23(3):135–41.

19. Siddiq MM, Chan AT, Miorin L, et al. Physiology of cardiomyocyte injury in COVID-19. medRxiv 2020;2020:11.

20. Bulfamante GP, Perrucci GL, Falleni M, et al. Evidence of SARS-CoV-2 transcriptional activity in cardiomyocytes of COVID-19 patients without clinical signs of cardiac involvement. Biomedicines 2020;8(12):626.

21. Wichmann D, Sperhake JP, Lütgehetmann M, et al. Autopsy findings and venous thromboembolism in patients with COVID-19: a Prospective cohort study. Ann Intern Med 2020;173(4):268–77.

22. Puntmann VO, Carerj ML, Wieters I, et al. Outcomes of cardiovascular magnetic resonance Imaging in patients Recently Recovered from coronavirus disease 2019 (COVID-19). JAMA Cardiol 2020;5(11):1265–73.

23. Haque R, Kan H, Finkel MS. Effects of cytokines and nitric oxide on myocardial E-C coupling. Basic Res Cardiol 1998;93(Suppl 1):86–94.

24. Lazzerini PE, Laghi-Pasini F, Bertolozzi I, et al. Systemic inflammation as a novel QT-prolonging risk factor in patients with Torsades de Pointes. Heart 2017;103:1821–9.

25. Zhabyeyev P, Oudit GY. Sickle cell disease, interleukin-18, and arrhythmias. Blood 2021;137(9):1138–9.

26. Tsai YN, Hsiao YW, Lin SF, et al. Proinflammatory cytokine modulates Intracellular calcium handling and Enhances ventricular arrhythmia susceptibility. Front Cardiovasc Med 2021;8:623510.

27. Di Biase L, Romero J, Zado ES, et al. Variant of ventricular outflow tract ventricular arrhythmias requiring ablation from multiple sites: Intramural origin. Heart Rhythm 2019;16(5):724–32.

28. Solaimanzadeh J, Freilich A, Sood MR. Ventricular tachycardia with epicardial and pericardial fibrosis 6 months after resolution of subclinical COVID-19: a case report. J Med Case Rep 2021;15(1):305.

29. Mitrani RD, Dabas N, Goldberger JJ. COVID-19 cardiac injury: implications for long-term surveillance and outcomes in survivors. Heart Rhythm 2020;17(11):1984–90.

30. Della Rocca DG, Magnocavallo M, Lavalle C, et al. Evidence of systemic endothelial injury and microthrombosis in hospitalized COVID-19 patients at different stages of the disease. J Thromb Thrombolysis 2021;51(3):571–6.

31. Pellegrini D, Kawakami R, Guagliumi G, et al. Microthrombi as a major cause of cardiac injury in COVID-19: a pathologic study. Circulation 2021;143(10):1031–42.

32. D'Ascenzo F, De Filippo O, Borin A, et al. Impact of COVID-19 pandemic and infection on in hospital survival for patients presenting with acute coronary syndromes: a multicenter registry. Int J Cardiol 2021;332:227–34.

33. Luqman N, Sung RJ, Wang CL, et al. Myocardial ischemia and ventricular fibrillation: pathophysiology and clinical implications. Int J Cardiol 2007;119(3):283–90.

34. Tazmini K, Frisk M, Lewalle A, et al. Hypokalemia Promotes arrhythmia by distinct mechanisms in atrial and ventricular myocytes. Circ Res 2020;126(7):889–906.

35. Sealy WC, Young WG Jr, Harris JS. Studies on cardiac arrest: the relationship of hypercapnia to ventricular fibrillation. J Thorac Surg 1954;28(5):447–62.

36. Gettes LS. Electrolyte abnormalities underlying lethal and ventricular arrhythmias. Circulation 1992;85(1 Suppl):I70–6.

37. Chen Q, Xu J, Gianni C, et al. Simple electrocardiographic criteria for rapid identification of wide QRS complex tachycardia: the new limb lead algorithm. Heart Rhythm 2020;17(3):431–8.

38. Schrezenmeier E, Dörner T. Mechanisms of action of hydroxychloroquine and chloroquine: implications for rheumatology. Nat Rev Rheumatol 2020;16(3):155–66.

39. Saleh M, Gabriels J, Chang D, et al. Effect of chloroquine, hydroxychloroquine, and azithromycin on the corrected QT interval in patients with SARS-CoV-2 infection. Circ Arrhythm Electrophysiol 2020;13(6):e008662.

40. Gasperetti A, Biffi M, Duru F, et al. Arrhythmic safety of hydroxychloroquine in COVID-19 patients from different clinical settings. Europace 2020;22(12):1855–63.

41. Zhang M, Xie M, Li S, et al. Electrophysiologic studies on the risks and potential mechanism underlying the Proarrhythmic nature of azithromycin. Cardiovasc Toxicol 2017;17(4):434–40.

42. Marmolejo-Murillo LG, Aréchiga-Figueroa IA, Moreno-Galindo EG, et al. Chloroquine blocks the Kir4.1 channels by an open-pore blocking mechanism. Eur J Pharmacol 2017;800:40–7.

43. Yang Z, Prinsen JK, Bersell KR, et al. Azithromycin causes a novel Proarrhythmic syndrome. Circ Arrhythm Electrophysiol 2017;10(4):e003560.

44. Chorin E, Wadhwani L, Magnani S, et al. QT interval prolongation and torsade de pointes in patients with COVID-19 treated with hydroxychloroquine/azithromycin. Heart Rhythm 2020;17:1425–33.

45. Romero J, Alviz I, Parides M, et al. T-wave inversion as a manifestation of COVID-19 infection: a case series. J Interv Card Electrophysiol 2020;59(3):485–93.
46. Lazzerini PE, Boutjdir M, Capecchi PL. COVID-19, arrhythmic risk, and inflammation: Mind the Gap. Circulation 2020;142(1):7–9.
47. Zylla MM, Merle U, Vey JA, et al. Predictors and Prognostic implications of cardiac arrhythmias in patients hospitalized for COVID-19. J Clin Med 2021; 10(1):133.
48. Gopinathannair R, Merchant FM, Lakkireddy DR, et al. COVID-19 and cardiac arrhythmias: a global perspective on arrhythmia characteristics and management strategies. J Interv Card Electrophysiol 2020;59(2):329–36.
49. Roedl K, Jarczak D, Drolz A, et al. Severe liver dysfunction complicating course of COVID-19 in the critically ill: multifactorial cause or direct viral effect? Ann Intensive Care 2021;11(1):44.
50. Ashrafian H, Davey P. Is amiodarone an underrecognized cause of acute respiratory failure in the ICU? Chest 2001;120(1):275–82.
51. Argyriou M, Hountis P, Antonopoulos N, et al. Acute fatal post-CABG low dose amiodarone lung toxicity. Asian Cardiovasc Thorac Ann 2007;15(6):e66–8.
52. Baumann H, Fichtenkamm P, Schneider T, et al. Rapid onset of amiodarone induced pulmonary toxicity after lung lobe resection - a case report and review of recent literature. Ann Med Surg (Lond) 2017;21:53–7.
53. Ott MC, Khoor A, Leventhal JP, et al. Pulmonary toxicity in patients receiving low-dose amiodarone. Chest 2003;123:646–51.
54. Terzo F, Ricci A, D'Ascanio M, et al. Amiodarone-induced pulmonary toxicity with an excellent response to treatment: a case report. Respir Med Case Rep 2019;29:100974.
55. Camus P, Martin WJ II, Rosenow EC III. Amiodarone pulmonary toxicity. Clin Chest Med 2004;25:65–75.
56. Tarantino N, Della Rocca DG, Faggioni M, et al. Epicardial ablation complications. Card Electrophysiol Clin 2020;12(3):409–18.
57. Hussain N, Bhattacharyya A, Prueksaritanond S. Amiodarone-induced cirrhosis of liver: what predicts mortality? ISRN Cardiol 2013;2013:617943.
58. Azraai M, McMahon M, Dick R. Case report of amiodarone-associated allergic pneumonitis amidst the COVID-19 pandemic. Rev Cardiovasc Med 2021;22(1):181–4.
59. Kow CS, Hasan SS. Amiodarone in COVID-19: let's not forget its potential for pulmonary toxicity. Eur J Prev Cardiol 2020. https://doi.org/10.1093/eurjpc/zwaa086. zwaa086.
60. Schmit G, Lelotte J, Vanhaebost J, et al. The liver in COVID-19-related death: Protagonist or Innocent Bystander? Pathobiology 2021;88(1):88–94.
61. Mitra RL, Greenstein SA, Epstein LM. An algorithm for managing QT prolongation in coronavirus disease 2019 (COVID-19) patients treated with either chloroquine or hydroxychloroquine in conjunction with azithromycin: possible benefits of intravenous lidocaine. Heartrhythm Case Rep 2020;6(5):244–8.
62. Stadler K, Ha HR, Ciminale V, et al. Amiodarone alters late endosomes and inhibits SARS coronavirus infection at a post-endosomal level. Am J Respir Cell Mol Biol 2008;39:142–9.
63. Ito H, Ono K, Nishio R, et al. Amiodarone inhibits interleukin 6 production and attenuates myocardial injury induced by viral myocarditis in mice. Cytokine 2002;17:197–202.
64. Ide T, Tsutsui H, Kinugawa S, et al. Amiodarone protects cardiac myocytes against oxidative injury by its free radical scavenging action. Circulation 1999; 100:690–2.
65. Castaldo N, Aimo A, Castiglione V, et al. Safety and efficacy of amiodarone in a patient with COVID-19. JACC Case Rep 2020;2(9):1307–10.
66. Sanchis-Gomar F, Lavie CJ, Morin DP, et al. Amiodarone in the COVID-19 Era: treatment for symptomatic patients only, or drug to prevent infection? Am J Cardiovasc Drugs 2020;20(5):413–8.
67. Available at: https://clinicaltrials.gov/ct2/show/NCT04351763. Accessed on July 5, 2021.
68. Cronin EM, Bogun FM, Maury P, et al. 2019 HRS/EHRA/APHRS/LAHRS expert consensus statement on catheter ablation of ventricular arrhythmias: Executive summary. J Arrhythm 2020;36(1):1–58.
69. Priori SG, Blomström-Lundqvist C, Mazzanti A, et al, ESC Scientific Document Group. 2015 ESC guidelines for the management of patients with ventricular arrhythmias and the prevention of sudden cardiac death: the task Force for the management of patients with ventricular arrhythmias and the prevention of sudden cardiac death of the European society of Cardiology (ESC). Endorsed by: association for European Paediatric and congenital Cardiology (AEPC). Eur Heart J 2015;36(41):2793–867.
70. Briceño DF, Romero J, Villablanca PA, et al. Long-term outcomes of different ablation strategies for ventricular tachycardia in patients with structural heart disease: systematic review and meta-analysis. Europace 2018;20(1):104–15.

COVID-19–Associated Endothelial Dysfunction and Microvascular Injury
From Pathophysiology to Clinical Manifestations

Maria Paola Canale, MD[a,b], Rossella Menghini, PhD[a],
Eugenio Martelli, MD[c,d], Massimo Federici, MD[a,b],*

KEYWORDS

- Covid-19 clinical manifestations • Endothelial dysfunction • Systemic inflammation • ACE2
- ADAM17

KEY POINTS

- The broad spectrum of clinical manifestations, affecting almost all organs and systems, is a consequence of the endothelial dysfunction and systemic inflammatory response.
- Endothelial cells activated by a hyperinflammatory state induced by viral infection may promote localized inflammation, increase reactive oxidative species production, and alter dynamic interplay between the procoagulant and fibrinolytic factors in the vascular system, leading to thrombotic disease not only in the pulmonary circulation but also in peripheral veins and arteries.
- Several data support the involvement of an increased activity of ADAM17 in both COVID-19's comorbidities and SARS-CoV-2 infection. In fact, the ADAM17 upregulation leads to the angiotensin-converting enzyme 2 (ACE2) ectodomain proteolytic cleavage, facilitating viral entry, and to the cleavage of tumor necrosis factor alpha and interleukin-6 receptor and other proinflammatory molecules, contributing to the "cytokine storm" and reinforcing the inflammatory process during SARS-CoV-2 infection.
- The molecular interaction of SARS-CoV-2 with the ACE2 receptor located in the endothelial cell surface, either at the pulmonary and systemic level, leads to early impairment of endothelial function, which, in turn, is followed by vascular inflammation and thrombosis of peripheral blood vessels.

INTRODUCTION

Coronavirus-19 disease (COVID-19) affects more people than previous coronavirus infections, namely severe acute respiratory syndrome (SARS) and middle east respiratory syndrome (MERS) and has a higher mortality. Higher incidence and mortality can probably be explained by COVID-19 causative agent's greater affinity (about 10–20 times) for angiotensin-converting enzyme 2 (ACE2) receptor compared with other coronaviruses.[1,2] According to the World Health Organization's (WHO) recent data "there have been 199.466.211 confirmed cases of COVID-19, including 4.244.541 deaths" (source: WHO data, August 4, 2021). In the same way as SARS and MERS, it affects the respiratory system. Nevertheless, because of the viral rapid diffusion and the increased numbers of infected people, many extra respiratory system manifestations have been

[a] Department of Systems Medicine, University of Rome Tor Vergata, Rome, Italy; [b] Center for Atherosclerosis, Policlinico Tor Vergata, Rome, Italy; [c] Department of General and Specialist Surgery "P. Stefanini", Sapienza University of Rome, Italy; [d] Division of Vascular Surgery, S. Anna and S. Sebastiano Hospital, Caserta, Italy
* Corresponding author. Department of Systems Medicine, Via Montpellier 1, Roma 00133, Italy.
E-mail address: federicm@uniroma2.it

Card Electrophysiol Clin 14 (2022) 21–28
https://doi.org/10.1016/j.ccep.2021.10.003
1877-9182/22/© 2021 Elsevier Inc. All rights reserved.

documented.[3–5] Severe symptoms result from hyperinflammatory response, which in turn causes systemic cytokine release and endothelial damage, and several clinical and laboratory findings support the role of endothelial dysfunction in the pathophysiology of disease, suggesting that the endothelium may represent an attractive target for new treatments.[6]

In this review, the authors first summarize clinical manifestations, then present symptoms of COVID-19 and the pathophysiological mechanisms underlying specific organ/system disease. After, they review current understanding of key pathophysiological mechanisms with particular regard to the role of endothelial dysfunction, microvascular injury, and systemic inflammatory response in disease progression and severity. Finally, they illustrate possible novel mechanisms and treatments aimed at protecting the endothelium.

COVID-19 CLINICAL MANIFESTATIONS

COVID-19 transmission mainly occurs directly via respiratory and saliva droplets from person to person. Indirect transmission, through fomites, may also occur. Airborne transmission only occurs when procedures generate aerosol. Incubation period is usually less than 1 week (about 5–6 days) but may last longer up to 2 weeks. Initial symptoms are nonspecific and similarly to other virosis such as influenza: fatigue, myalgias, dry cough, and low-grade fever.[7] Symptoms improve in most of the cases or progress to dyspnea in fewer ones.[3] Zeng and colleagues reviewed the symptomatology of COVID-19: the commonest signs/symptoms were fever (90%) and cough (68%) followed by dyspnea (22%), headache (12%), and sore throat (14%). Diarrhea was present in only about 4% of patients. Mean duration of fever in survivors is about 12 days, whereas mean duration of cough is slightly longer (19 days).[8] Although fever is a very common finding, its absence does not rule out the diagnosis.[9] Longer duration of fever is proportionate to disease's severity (31 days for patients admitted to the intensive care unit vs 9 days for those hospitalized in a different setting)[10]. As mentioned earlier, in about one-fifth of patients disease progresses to dyspnea.[3,7] Rapid progression to respiratory failure requiring noninvasive and invasive ventilation may occur. Viral respiratory invasion alone is insufficient to explain these findings. Endothelial dysfunction, subsequent inflammation, and lung injury with diffuse alveolar damage leading in some cases to acute distress respiratory syndrome is the underlying pathophysiological

mechanism responsible for respiratory failure.[7] Patients may experience other clinical features that strongly suggest endothelial dysfunction and microvascular thrombosis. Pain, warmth, and localized limb swelling are consistent with deep venous thrombosis, and acute onset tachycardia, dyspnea, and chest pain strongly suggest pulmonary embolism.[5]

The alterations of the coagulation mechanisms observed in COVID-19 can lead to acute thrombotic phenomena of the arteries of the lower limbs, curiously even in patients with healthy arteries (ie, in the absence of underlying peripheral arterial disease) or without atrial fibrillation or preexisting coagulation disorders. The most severe acute ischemia occurs in patients admitted to intensive care units for severe forms of COVID-19 pneumonia: they rarely represent the only clinical manifestation of the infection. The conservative approach with medical therapy alone may be the most appropriate, considering the poor results of surgical revascularization. This latter, on the contrary, has always been characterized by excellent results in non-COVID patients operated on within a few hours of the onset of acute symptoms. The rate of limb loss/amputation is dramatically high in patients with COVID affected by acute limb ischemia.[11]

Concomitant oliguria and general symptoms (ie, nausea and vomiting) deserve urgent renal function testing and raise the possibility of uremia in the setting of acute kidney injury. In addition, new-onset generalized edema reflects heart failure and/or heavy proteinuria. Moreover, the presence/absence of associated signs/symptoms may further contribute to orient the diagnosis during patient's physical examination. For instance, the coexistence of dyspnea, new-onset generalized edema with symmetric periorbital involvement, and negative hepatojugular reflux indicates concomitant respiratory and renal rather than cardiac involvement. Laboratory tests would eventually show abnormal renal function, hypoalbuminemia, and heavy proteinuria, and transthoracic echocardiography confirms normal systolic function and absence of valves abnormalities. Severe headache may reflect central venous thrombosis or intracerebral hemorrhage. Finally, systemic inflammatory response may indirectly cause neurologic signs/symptoms such as headache, encephalopathy, or seizures.[5]

COVID-19 is characterized by a wide spectrum of clinical severity. Asymptomatic persons experience no symptoms and have normal chest radiographs but play an important role in disease transmission to others. Mild illness is characterized by general symptoms common to other virosis; gastrointestinal symptoms may be present too (abdominal pain, nausea, vomiting, and diarrhea). In moderate illness, symptoms of pneumonia are present with still normal blood gases, and interstitial ground-glass opacities appear on high-resolution computed tomography scan. Severe illness is characterized by pneumonia with hypoxemia (peripheral oxygen saturation is <92% in ambient air). Finally, critical state is characterized by the presence of acute distress respiratory syndrome, coagulation disorders, cardiac failure, acute renal injury, and shock.[7,9,12–17] Patients with comorbidities have a worse disease course and prognosis compared with healthy ones, as observed in previous coronavirus infections.[1] Advanced age, male sex, diabetes, hypertension, ischemic heart disease, cancer, chronic obstructive pulmonary disease, and chronic renal insufficiency are risk factors for developing a severe form of COVID-19.[18–20] These conditions affect negatively patient's immune system.[1,21]

A full description of the COVID-19 treatment by organ/system involvement is beyond the scope of this review. Most suitable treatment should be prescribed depending on disease's severity and organ involvement. At the present time, treatment encompasses oxygen (when required); symptomatic, antiinflammatory, antiviral, and anticoagulant drugs (prophylactic or therapeutic, with low-molecular-weight heparin); and monoclonal antibodies. Moreover, in selected patients resistant to treatment, plasma exchange therapy and immunomodulatory medications may be required.[7] Updated COVID-19 treatment guidelines by disease's severity are provided by national and international institutions at their Web sites. Finally, major concern has been raised about the use of renin-angiotensin blocking agents in patients with COVID-19. Routine discontinuation is not recommended by the guidelines of international cardiology societies.[22,23]

A Molecular Perspective to Explain Endothelial Cell Activation in COVID 19

The COVID-19 clinical manifestations by organ/system and the underlying pathophysiological mechanisms of disease are summarized in **Tables 1–3**. Mechanisms that specifically contribute to determine a clinical manifestation are also

---

Table 1
COVID-19 clinical manifestations by system and pathophysiological mechanism

Clinical Manifestations (Refs.[1–5])	Pathophysiological Mechanisms (Refs.[1–5])
Respiratory Pneumonia Acute respiratory distress syndrome Microvascular lung thrombosis Respiratory failure	*Multifactorial* Direct viral injury and inflammation Endothelial dysfunction • proinflammatory • procoagulant • proaggregating • capillary leakage • increased vascular permeability Systemic inflammatory response ("cytokine storm")
Cardiac Myocarditis/pericarditis Arrhythmias Right or/and left heart failure Acute coronary syndrome Cardiogenic shock	*Multifactorial* Direct viral injury and inflammation Endothelial dysfunction • proinflammatory • procoagulant High ACE2 levels Systemic inflammatory response ("cytokine storm") Hypoxemia Oxygen supply mismatch

Arterial
Large vessel occlusion: clinical presentation
  depending on the affected artery
  (cerebral, cardiac, mesenteric, renal, limb)
Central nervous system vasculitis
	Multifactorial
	Direct viral injury
	Endothelial dysfunction
	• proinflammatory
	• procoagulant
	• proaggregating
	Hypoxia

Table 2
COVID-19 clinical manifestations by system and pathophysiological mechanism

Clinical Manifestations (Refs.[1–5])	Pathophysiological Mechanisms (Refs.[1–5])

Venous thromboembolism
  Deep vein thrombosis
  Pulmonary embolism
  Intravenous/intraarterial catheters and
    extracorporeal circuit thrombosis
  Central venous thrombosis
	Multifactorial
	Endothelial dysfunction
	• proinflammatory
	• prooxidant
	• procoagulant
	• proaggregating
	Hypoxia

Renal
  Hematuria/proteinuria
  Electrolyte abnormalities
  Acute tubular necrosis
  Acute kidney injury
	Multifactorial
	Direct viral injury
	Endothelial dysfunction leading to
	• vasoconstriction
	• microvascular dysfunction
	Systemic inflammatory response ("cytokine storm")
	Immune complexes
	Hypovolemia

Hepatic/Gastrointestinal
  Liver function tests abnormalities
  Gastrointestinal symptoms (diarrhea,
    abdominal pain, nausea, vomiting)
	Multifactorial
	Direct viral injury
	Endothelial dysfunction
	• proinflammatory
	• procoagulant
	• proaggregating
	Microvascular small bowel injury
	Systemic inflammatory response ("cytokine storm")
	Hypoxia-associated metabolic abnormalities

Neurologic/ocular
  Ageusia, anosmia
  Dizziness, headache, seizures
  Guillain-Barré syndrome
  Encephalitis/meningoencephalitis
  Encephalomyelitis
  Acute hemorrhagic necrotizing
    encephalopathy
  Conjunctivitis and retinal changes
	Multifactorial
	Direct nervous system invasion for ageusia, anosmia, encephalitis, meningoencephalitis
	Direct viral injury
	Endothelial dysfunction
	• proinflammatory
	• procoagulant
	Systemic inflammatory response ("cytokine storm")
	Postinfectious/immune-mediated for Guillain-Barré syndrome, encephalomyelitis, acute hemorrhagic-necrotizing encephalopathy
	Direct viral injury and inflammation for conjunctivitis

reported. Endothelium represents an interface between blood and body's tissues.[24] The broad spectrum of clinical manifestations, affecting almost all organs and systems, is a consequence of the endothelial dysfunction and systemic inflammatory response. As shown in **Tables 1–3**, endothelial dysfunction's different components and systemic inflammatory response, namely "cytokine storm," play a pivotal role in determining most of the clinical manifestations of COVID-19 (left column) and always underlie severe manifestations.[4,5]

Recent findings suggest that endothelial dysfunction represents a crucial pathologic characteristic in COVID19, being implicated in microvascular and macrovascular complications associated with the infection, including myocardial infarction and stroke.[25] Biomarkers of endothelial dysfunction are increased in patients with COVID-19 and are associated with more severe

Table 3
COVID-19 clinical manifestations by system and pathophysiological mechanism

Clinical Manifestations (Refs.[1–5])	Pathophysiological Mechanisms (Refs.[1–5])
Dermatologic Acrocutaneous lesions Erythematous and maculopapular rash Vesicles Livedoid, necrotic lesions, petechiae	*Multifactorial* Endothelial dysfunction with deposition of microthrombi Systemic inflammatory response ("cytokine storm") Immune response sensitivity Vasculitis
Hematologic Blood cell count abnormalities (lymphopenia, leukocytosis neutrophilia, thrombocytopenia) Increased inflammatory markers Increased coagulation markers	*Multifactorial* Direct viral injury and inflammation and endothelial dysfunction proinflammatory for lymphopenia Systemic inflammatory response and/or bacterial infection for leukocytosis Systemic inflammatory response (early phase) for increased inflammatory markers and increased coagulation makers
Miscellaneous Fever Fatigue Myalgias Endocrine (new-onset diabetes, severe illness in diabetic/obese patients, ketoacidosis) High-grade fever Hypotension Multiorgan dysfunction Disseminated intravascular coagulation Long-term COVID-19 syndrome	Cytokine release common to other virus for fever, fatigue, and myalgias Direct viral injury, lactate level increase, low oxygen, and low pH for myalgias Multifactorial for endocrine Endothelial dysfunction leading to systemic inflammatory response ("cytokine storm") ACE2 viral binding on beta cells Impaired counter-regulation (not specific to COVID-19) Altered immune response (not specific to COVID-19) Systemic inflammatory response for high-grade fever, hypotension, and multiorgan dysfunction Endothelial dysfunction leading to coagulation/fibrinolytic abnormalities, macro- and microthrombosis, bleeding for disseminated intravascular coagulation Multifactorial for long-term COVID Virus-specific pathophysiologic changes Inflammatory damage and immunologic aberrations Sequelae of postcritical illness

forms of the disease and high mortality.[26] Endothelial dysfunction may result from a combination of direct viral effects, as suggested by the presence of viral elements within the endothelium in autopsies from patients who died of COVID19, and a consequence of virus-dependent activation of inflammatory response.[27] Moreover, endothelial changes are multiorgan, indicating that endothelial dysfunction may be involved in numerous symptoms of SARS-CoV-2-positive patients.[28] Injury of endothelial cells is involved in several pathophysiological mechanisms that may promote the occurrence of micro- and macrovascular involvement in COVID19 infection. Endothelial cells activated by a hyperinflammatory state induced by viral infection may promote localized inflammation, increase reactive oxidative species production, and alter dynamic interplay between the procoagulant and fibrinolytic factors in the vascular system, leading to thrombotic disease not only in the pulmonary circulation but also in peripheral veins and arteries.[29] It was proposed that mitochondrial dysfunction and oxidative stress, induced by viral infection, can initiate a feedback loop, promoting a chronic state of inflammatory cytokine production and endothelial alteration even after the viral particles have been eliminated from the body.[30] Agents that limit endothelial dysfunction may mitigate the proinflammatory and prothrombotic state induced by COVID-19 infection; therefore, targeted inhibition of cytokines, major effectors of endothelial activation, represents a more focused approach than generalized antiinflammatory agents. Some clinical trials that use strategies aimed to have inhibit the inflammasome–interleukin-1β (IL-1β)–IL-6 pathway already yielded preliminary results; some, but not all, indicate signals of efficacy being a critical aspect in the maintaining of the balance between the potential benefits versus the potential of lowering immunologic defences.[24]

ADAM17 Abridges COVID19 and Endothelial Dysfunction

ADAM17 (a disintegrin and a metalloproteinase 17) is a type I transmembrane protein that belongs to a superfamily of Zn-dependent metalloproteases. ADAM17 plays a key role in the regulation of the proteolytic release from cellular membranes of some cytokines, chemokines, growth factors, and their receptors, affecting downstream signaling and cellular responses. Increased ADAM17-mediated shedding has been described in a variety of diseases such as ischemia, heart failure, arthritis, atherosclerosis, diabetes, cancer, neurologic, and immune diseases. Tissue inhibitor of metalloproteinase 3 (TIMP3), a key endogenous inhibitor involved in regulation of the activity of matrix metalloproteinases and ADAMs, is the only known physiologic inhibitor of ADAM17. Previous reports have implicated the ADAM17/TIMP3 dyad as a mediator between metabolic stimuli, inflammation, and innate immunity.[31] The increased activity of ADAM17 has been correlated with increased insulin resistance and hyperglycemia. Furthermore, the upregulation of ADAM17 activity increased insulin receptor resistance in patients with type 2 diabetes.[32] Several data support the involvement of an increased activity of ADAM17 in both COVID-19's comorbidities and SARS-CoV-2 infection. In fact, the ADAM17 upregulation leads to the ACE2 ectodomain proteolytic cleavage, facilitating viral entry, and to the cleavage of tumor necrosis factor alpha and IL-6R and other proinflammatory molecules, contributing to the "cytokine storm" and reinforcing the inflammatory process during SARS-CoV-2 infection. This hyperinflammatory state has deleterious effects on the vascular system with resulting endothelial cell dysfunction and not only affects local

endothelial function but can also provoke a prothrombotic and antifibrinolytic imbalance in blood that favors thrombus accumulation.[33] Coagulation abnormalities and disruption of factors released by endothelial cells represent also the common pathophysiological link between SARS-CoV-2 infection and the cardiovascular events, including acute cardiac injury, stroke, heart failure, arrhythmias, and cardiomyopathies. In particular, the molecular interaction of SARS-CoV-2 with the ACE2 receptor located in the endothelial cell surface, either at the pulmonary and systemic level, leads to early impairment of endothelial function, which, in turn, is followed by vascular inflammation and thrombosis of peripheral blood vessels.[34]

In this context, the worse clinical outcome observed in patients with COVID-19 with diabetes may be in part related to the increased ADAM17 activity and its unbalanced interplay with ACE2. Therefore, strategies aimed to inhibit ADAM17 activity may be explored to develop new effective therapeutic approaches.

SUMMARY

In the last 2 years a great progress had been made to provide mechanisms explaining how Sars-COV-2 affects human health. Data point to endothelium as a major site of action of the virus. The overactivation of the physiologic functions of endothelium such as control of vasomotion, vascular permeability, fibrinolysis and hemostasis, inflammation, and oxidative stress may contribute to the COVID19 disease and provide a framework to develop new therapeutics against Sars-COV-2 in the future.

CLINICS CARE POINTS

- Endothelial dysfunction represents a crucial pathologic characteristic in COVID19, being implicated in microvascular and macrovascular complications associated with the infection, including myocardial infarction and stroke.
- Endothelial dysfunction may result from a combination of direct viral effects, as suggested by the presence of viral elements within the endothelium in autopsies from patients who died of COVID19, and a consequence of virus-dependent activation of inflammatory response.
- Treatment encompasses oxygen (when required); symptomatic, antiinflammatory, antiviral, and anticoagulant drugs (prophylactic or therapeutic, with low-molecular-weight heparin), and monoclonal antibodies.

CONFLICTS OF INTEREST/DISCLOSURES

This work was in part supported by PRIN 2017FM74HK (to M.F.).

REFERENCES

1. Johnson KD, Harris C, Cain JK, et al. Pulmonary and extra-pulmonary clinical manifestations of COVID-19. Front Med (Lausanne) 2020;7:526.
2. Wrapp D, Wang N, Corbett KS, et al. Cryo-EM structure of the 2019-nCoV spike in the prefusion conformation. Science 2020;367:1260–3.
3. Canatan D, Vives Corrons JL, De Sanctis V. The multifacets of COVID-19 in adult patients: a concise clinical review on pulmonary and extrapulmonary manifestations for healthcare physicians. Acta Biomed 2020;91:e2020173.
4. Gupta A, Madhavan MV, Sehgal K, et al. Extrapulmonary manifestations of COVID-19. Nat Med 2020;26:1017–32.
5. Gavriilaki E, Anyfanti P, Gavriilaki M, et al. Endothelial dysfunction in COVID-19: lessons learned from coronaviruses. Curr Hypertens Rep 2020;22:63.
6. Castro P, Palomo M, Moreno-Castaño AB, et al. Is the endothelium the missing link in the pathophysiology and treatment of COVID-19 complications? Cardiovasc Drugs Ther 2021;1–14.
7. Parasher A. COVID-19: current understanding of its pathophysiology, clinical presentation and treatment. Postgrad Med J 2021;97:312–20.
8. Zheng J. SARS-CoV-2: an emerging coronavirus that causes a global threat. Int J Biol Sci 2020;16:1678–85.
9. Guan WJ, Ni ZY, Hu Y, et al. China medical treatment expert group for Covid-19. Clinical characteristics of coronavirus disease 2019 in China. N Engl J Med 2020;382:1708–20.
10. Chen J, Qi T, Liu L, et al. Clinical progression of patients with COVID-19 in Shanghai, China. J Infect 2020;80:e1–6.
11. Etkin Y, Conway AM, Silpe J, et al. Acute arterial thromboembolism in patients with COVID-19 in the New York City Area. Ann Vasc Surg 2021;70:290–4.
12. Li Q, Guan X, Wu P, et al. Early transmission dynamics in Wuhan, China, of novel coronavirus-infected pneumonia. N Engl J Med 2020;382:1199–207.
13. Yuki K, Fujiogi M, Koutsogiannaki S. COVID-19 pathophysiology: a review. Clin Immunol 2020;215:108427.
14. Donnelly CA, Ghani AC, Leung GM, et al. Epidemiological determinants of spread of causal agent of severe acute respiratory syndrome in Hong Kong. Lancet 2003;361:1761–6.
15. Goyal P, Choi JJ, Pinheiro LC, et al. Clinical characteristics of covid-19 in New York City. N Engl J Med 2020;382:2372–4.
16. Young BE, Ong SWX, Kalimuddin S, et al. Singapore 2019 Novel coronavirus outbreak research team. epidemiologic features and clinical course of patients infected with SARS-CoV-2 in Singapore. JAMA 2020;323:1488–94.
17. Cheung KS, Hung IFN, Chan PPY, et al. Gastrointestinal manifestations of SARS-CoV-2 infection and virus load in fecal samples from a Hong Kong Cohort: systematic review and meta-analysis. Gastroenterology 2020;159:81–95.
18. Liu X, Zhou H, Zhou Y, et al. Risk factors associated with disease severity and length of hospital stay in COVID-19 patients. J Infect 2020;81:e95–7.
19. Wynants L, Van Calster B, Collins GS, et al. Prediction models for diagnosis and prognosis of covid-19: systematic review and critical appraisal. BMJ 2020;369:m1328.
20. Pijls BG, Jolani S, Atherley A, et al. Demographic risk factors for COVID-19 infection, severity, ICU admission and death: a meta-analysis of 59 studies. BMJ Open 2021;11:e044640.
21. Park J, Lee DS, Christakis NA, et al. The impact of cellular networks on disease comorbidity. Mol Syst Biol 2009;5:262.
22. European Society of Cardiology Position statement of the ESC Council on hypertension on ACE-Inhibitors and angiotensin receptor blockers. Eur Heart J 2021 Nov 16;ehab696. https://doi.org/10.1093/eurheartj/ehab696.
23. Bozkurt B, Kovacs R, Harrington B. Joint HFSA/ACC/AHA statement Addresses concerns Re: Using RAAS Antagonists in COVID-19. J Card Fail 2020;26:370.
24. Libby P, Lüscher T. COVID-19 is, in the end, an endothelial disease. Eur Heart J 2020;41:3038–44.
25. Gu SX, Tyagi T, Jain K, et al. Thrombocytopathy and endotheliopathy: crucial contributors to COVID-19 thromboinflammation. Nat Rev Cardiol 2021;18:194–209.
26. Pine AB, Meizlish ML, Goshua G, et al. Circulating markers of angiogenesis and endotheliopathy in COVID-19. Pulm Circ 2020;10. 204589402096654.
27. Varga Z, Flammer AJ, Steiger P, et al. Endothelial cell infection and endotheliitis in COVID-19. Lancet 2020;395:1417–8.
28. Fodor A, Tiperciuc B, Login C, et al. Endothelial dysfunction, inflammation, and oxidative stress in COVID-19-mechanisms and therapeutic targets. Oxid Med Cell Longev 2021;2021:8671713.
29. Siddiqi HK, Libby P, Ridker PM. COVID-19 - a vascular disease. Trends Cardiovasc Med 2021;31:1–5.
30. Chang R R, Mamun A A, Dominic A A, et al. SARSCoV-2 mediated endothelial dysfunction: the potential role of chronic oxidative stress. Front Physiol 2021;11:605908.
31. Menghini R, Fiorentino L, Casagrande V, et al. The role of ADAM17 in metabolic inflammation. Atherosclerosis 2013;228:12–7.

32. Cardellini M, Menghini R, Luzi A, et al. Decreased IRS2 and TIMP3 expression in monocytes from offspring of type 2 diabetic patients is correlated with insulin resistance and increased intima-media thickness. Diabetes 2011;60:3265–70.

33. Zipeto D, Palmeira JDF, Argañaraz GA, et al. ACE2/ ADAM17/TMPRSS2 interplay may be the main risk factor for COVID-19. Front Immunol 2020;11: 576745.

34. Maiuolo J, Mollace R, Gliozzi M, et al. The contribution of endothelial dysfunction in systemic injury subsequent to SARS-Cov-2 infection. Int J Mol Sci 2020;21:9309.

COVID-19, Acute Myocardial Injury, and Infarction

Armando Del Prete, MD[a,b,]*, Francesca Conway, MD[c],
Domenico G. Della Rocca, MD, PhD[d], Giuseppe Biondi-Zoccai, MD, MStat[a,e,f],
Francesco De Felice, MD[g], Carmine Musto, MD, PhD[g], Marco Picichè, MD[h],
Eugenio Martuscelli, MD, PhD[i], Andrea Natale, MD[d,j,k],
Francesco Versaci, MD[a]

KEYWORDS

- COVID-19 • Myocardial injury • Myocardial infarction • SARS-CoV-2

KEY POINTS

- Severe acute respiratory syndrome coronavirus-2 (SARS-CoV-2) primarily infects the respiratory tract but can broadly affect the cardiovascular system too.
- SARS-CoV-2 can damage the myocardium by direct viral invasion or indirectly through inflammation, endothelial activation, and microvascular thrombosis.
- Myocardial injury affects about one-quarter of patients with COVID-19, even those without prior cardiovascular disease.
- Patients with COVID-19 who experience myocardial injury have higher hospital mortality rates and can present long-term complications.
- The diagnosis of myocardial injury can be particularly challenging in the context of COVID-19, particularly in patients with advanced disease.

INTRODUCTION

The new coronavirus-associated disease 2019 (COVID-19), due to severe acute respiratory syndrome coronavirus-2 (SARS-CoV-2), represents an unprecedented public health emergency that has been accompanied by a global health crisis. Although SARS-CoV-2 primarily infects the respiratory system, causing a variety of clinical presentations, from asymptomatic infection to interstitial pneumonia and severe acute respiratory distress syndrome (ARDS), the cardiovascular implications are also significant, especially in their contribution to disease morbidity and mortality.

When the cardiovascular system is affected, complications can include myocardial injury, acute myocardial infarction (MI), heart failure, myocarditis, dysrhythmias, and venous thromboembolic events.[1] Although various studies have demonstrated an association between preexisting

[a] Division of Cardiology, Santa Maria Goretti Hospital, Via Guido Reni 1, 04100 Latina, Italy; [b] Department of Systems Medicine, University of Rome "Tor Vergata", Via Montpellier 1, 00133 Rome, Italy; [c] London School of Hygiene and Tropical Medicine, Keppel St, London WC1E 7HT, United Kingdom; [d] Texas Cardiac Arrhythmia Institute, St. David's Medical Center, 000 N Interstate Hwy 35 Suite 720, Austin, TX 78705, USA; [e] Department of Medical-Surgical Sciences and Biotechnologies, Sapienza University, Corso della Repubblica 79, 04100 Latina, Italy; [f] Mediterranea Cardiocentro, Via Ponte di Tappia 82, 80133 Naples, Italy; [g] Division of Cardiology, San Camillo Hospital, Circonvallazione Gianicolense 87, 00152 Rome, Italy; [h] Department of Cardiac Surgery, San Bortolo Hospital, Viale Ferdinando Rodolfi 37, 36100 Vicenza, Italy; [i] Department of Biomedicine and Prevention, University of Rome "Tor Vergata", Via Montpellier 1, 00133 Rome, Italy; [j] Interventional Electrophysiology, Scripps Clinic, 9898 Genesee Ave Fl 3, La Jolla, CA 92037, USA; [k] Metro Health Medical Center, Case Western Reserve University School of Medicine, 9501 Euclid Ave, Cleveland, OH 44106, USA
* Corresponding author. Division of Cardiology, Santa Maria Goretti Hospital, Via Guido Reni 1, Latina, Italy.
E-mail address: armando.delprete85@gmail.com

Card Electrophysiol Clin 14 (2022) 29–39
https://doi.org/10.1016/j.ccep.2021.10.004
1877-9182/22/© 2021 Elsevier Inc. All rights reserved.

cardiovascular disease and severe COVID-19 manifestations, it is possible that the viral infection itself may lead to cardiac complications or exacerbate preexisting cardiovascular conditions.[2,3]

Acute myocardial injury is not uncommon in patients with COVID-19 and correlates with disease severity.[4] In addition, patients with long-term coronary artery disease or risk factors for atherosclerotic disease are at heightened risk of acute coronary syndromes (ACS) if infected with SARS-CoV-2. Acute coronary events in patients with COVID-19 may be the result of the systemic inflammatory hyperactivity, triggered by the viral infection and mediated by circulating cytokines that interact with preexisting atherosclerotic plaques, potentially causing plaque instability and rupture, ultimately leading to a type 1 MI.[5] In patients who eventually overcome myocardial injury and SARS-CoV-2 infection, there is evidence of long-term cardiovascular complications, although the magnitude of these sequelae is still unclear.

PHYSIOPATHOLOGICAL INVOLVEMENT OF THE CARDIOVASCULAR SYSTEM

SARS-CoV-2 primarily infects cells in the respiratory tract, causing a wide spectrum of respiratory manifestations, from asymptomatic or mild infection to bilateral interstitial pneumonia and severe ARDS.[1] There is also evidence supporting the affinity of the virus for multiple tissues, suggesting that SARS-CoV-2 has an organotropism that extends beyond the respiratory system, involving the brain, the liver, the kidney, and the cardiovascular district.[6] When the cardiovascular system is affected a vast range of complications can occur, from myocardial injury and acute MI to heart failure, myocarditis, dysrhythmias, and venous thromboembolic events.[1]

Previously published reports have described increased incidence of myocardial injury among patients with COVID-19.[7] During SARS-COV-2 infection the myocardium may be damaged by the viral invasion of cardiac muscle cells, inflammation and production of free radicals and reactive oxygen species, microvascular thrombosis, and a disproportion between oxygen supply and demand.[8] As a result, myocardial dysfunction, heart failure, myocardial injury, and both type 1 and type 2 MI may manifest, mediated by these one or more of these underlying mechanisms. Cardiac tissue tropism of SARS-CoV-2 is supported by the findings of an autopsy series of 20 patients: detectable viral SARS-CoV genome was found in 7 of the 20 heart samples, along with increased myocardial fibrosis and inflammation.[9]

Direct viral invasion is not the only mechanism through which SARS-CoV-2 can damage the heart.

A particularly interesting interaction has been described between SARS-CoV-2 and the renin angiotensin system (RAS).[10] The main hypothesis is that the RAS may be involved in the pathophysiology of COVID-19 via activation of the classic pathway. The angiotensin-converting enzyme 2 (ACE2) serves as a master regulator of the RAS. By metabolizing the vasoconstricting and proinflammatory angiotensin II (Ang II), ACE2 generates Ang 1 to 7, which counteracts the proinflammatory and prooxidant effects of Ang II.[11] Molecular studies have demonstrated that ACE2 is the SARS-CoV-2 cell entry receptor, through the activation of the viral outer membrane spike protein S by transmembrane protease serine 2 (TMPRSS2).[12] SARS-CoV-2 uses ACE2 as the port of entry by binding the extracellular domain of the host receptor through the S1/s2 subunits of the transmembrane spike glycoprotein.[13,14] Once a cell becomes infected with SARS-CoV-2, ACE2 is internalized, the virus can enter the cell and release its RNA to initiate replication and transcription of the viral genome. After synthesis and assembly of structural proteins, new virus is released from the cell by exocytosis, whereas host cells may be disabled or destroyed in the process.[15] Beyond causing direct cell damage through viral infiltration, SARS-CoV-2 downregulates ACE 2 expression and Ang 1 to 7 production, leading to the loss of the RAS counterregulatory protective arm.[16] By hampering the expression of ACE2, the beneficial degradation of Ang II to the counterregulatory Ang^{1-7} decreases, leading to unopposed Ang II effects, mediated by the receptor AT1. The AngII/AT1 activation yields several unfavorable effects, which include vasoconstrictive effects, but also host potentially detrimental effects on the endothelium, inflammation, and coagulation, ultimately increasing vascular permeability and promoting organ damage (**Fig. 1**).[17,18] These findings are supported by the fact that COVID-19 patients often present with increased AngII levels.[19,20] ACE2 is widely expressed in the lung but can also be found in high concentrations in the circulatory system at the level of arterial and venous endothelium as well as largely expressed by myocardial pericytes.[21,22]

Cardiovascular damage mediated by SARS-CoV-2 may therefore be the result of 3 different pathways:

- Direct myocardial damage due to viral entry through ACE2, resulting in myocardial cell destruction and inflammation;
- Indirect injury due to ACE2 downregulation following viral replication, with subsequent hyperactivation of the Ang II/AT1 system, responsible of vasoconstrictive, proinflammatory, and prooxidant effects

SARS-CoV-2 Infection & RAS Dysregulation

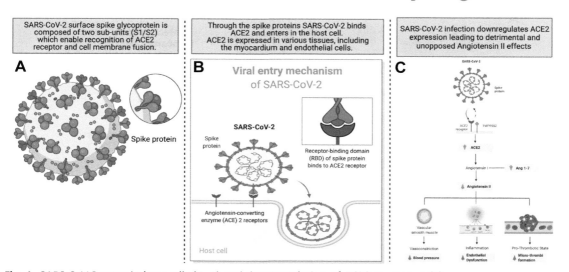

Fig. 1. SARS-CoV-2 entry in host cells (*A*, *B*) and downregulation of ACE2 expression (*C*).

- Indirect injury through the activation of B and T immune cells, leading to a systemic inflammatory response and increased cardiac stress due to hypoxemia.[23,24]

The immune-mediated pathway can generate a cytokine storm with high circulating levels of interleukin-2 (IL-2), IL-7, IL-10, and tumor necrosis factor, as a result of alternate immune response. This mechanism has been observed in severe forms of COVID-19 and can mediate myocardial injury as well as lung injury (particularly diffuse alveolar damage), finally leading to multiorgan failure. Components of the systemic inflammatory response can exert a negative inotropic effect, promote cardiomyocyte apoptosis and fibrosis, and induce the release of procoagulant factors.[25] The high plasma levels of activated macrophages that usually accompany conditions of hypercytokinemia can lead to further release of cytokines, including IL-1β and IL-6, which promote the expression of adhesion molecules, inflammatory cell infiltration, and vascular inflammation, contributing to formation and propagation of microcirculatory lesions and endothelial dysfunction.[26] Macrophages can also release procoagulant factors, further accelerating inflammation and augmenting a prothrombotic condition and thrombotic microangiopathy.[27] High circulating levels of macrophages might also interact with preexisting atherosclerotic plaques, leading to rupture of the fibrous cap and possibly causing type 1 MI.[28] These pathways are not unique to SARS-CoV-2, as viral infections are known to determine adverse cardiovascular events by precipitating plaque rupture in the setting of inflammation and a prothrombotic state.[29] It is also possible that hyperinflammation may generate a supply-demand mismatch at the level of the myocardium. SARS-CoV-2 infection can therefore precipitate myocardial injury by determining an oxygen supply–demand imbalance, either with or without acute coronary plaque pathology (type 1 and 2 MI).

SARS-CoV-2 can attack the cardiovascular system through different strategies: through direct damage of myocytes mediated by the virus as well as indirect mechanisms due to RAS pathway dysregulation, hyperinflammation leading to endothelial disfunction in different districts, and activation of procoagulant factors with microvascular thrombosis and oxygen supply–demand imbalance (**Fig. 2**). These mechanisms can take place in the presence of preexisting cardiovascular conditions or in patients without a clinical history of cardiovascular disease (CVD). Nonetheless, individuals with cardiovascular comorbidities or diabetes are at greater risk of experiencing a more aggressive SARS-CoV2 infection and the related cardiovascular complications.[30]

PREVALENCE AND CLINICAL OUTCOME OF MYOCARDIAL INJURY IN COVID-19

The detection of least one elevated cardiac troponin value greater than the 99th percentile upper reference limit defines myocardial injury. Although MI represents a manifestation of

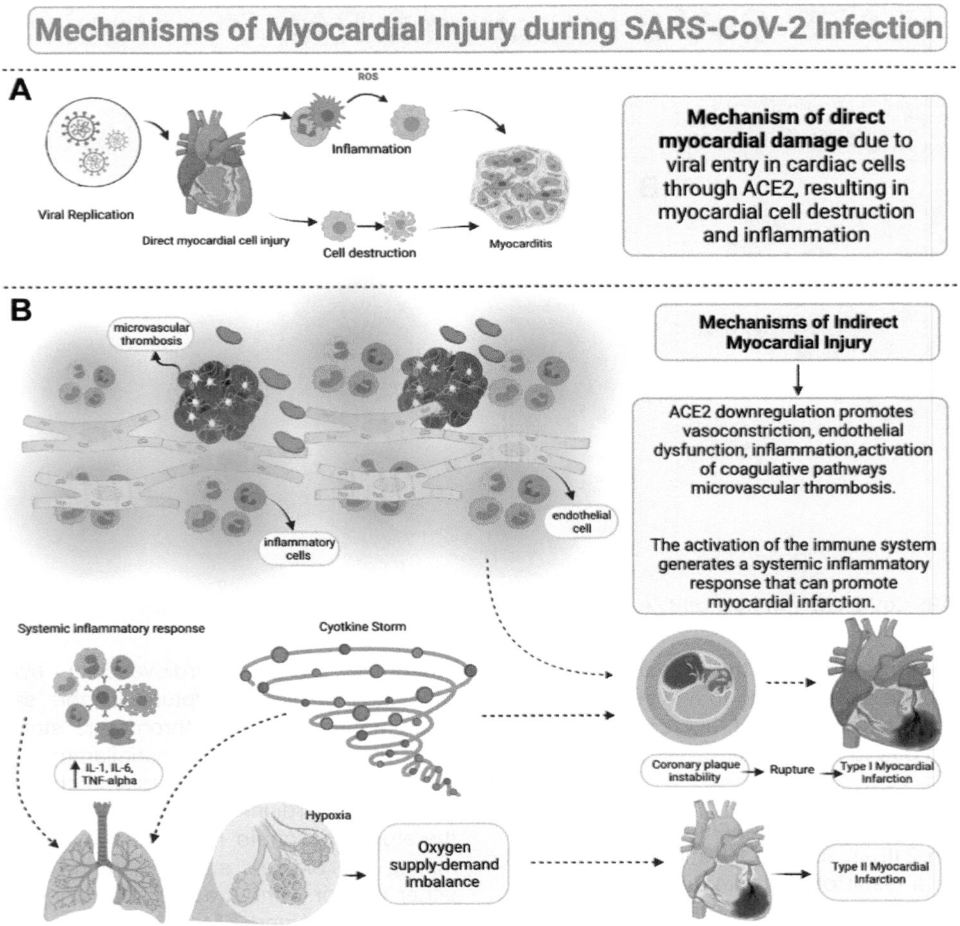

Fig. 2. Direct (*A*) and indirect (*B*) mechanisms of acute myocardial injury during SARS-CoV-2 infection and clinical outcomes.

myocardial injury, it requires clinical evidence of acute myocardial ischemia in order to perform the diagnosis. There are various subtypes of MI, the most common being type 1 infarction (characterized by plaque rupture, ulceration, erosion, or dissection resulting in coronary thrombosis) and type 2 infarction (secondary to myocardial oxygen supply–demand mismatch in the absence of coronary thrombosis).[31] Individuals infected with SARS-CoV-2 seem to be in a condition of increased susceptibility to various forms of myocardial injury.[32]

A study conducted in Wuhan showed evidence of cardiac damage with high levels of circulating troponin in up to 28% of patients with SARS-CoV-2. Furthermore, patients with evidence of cardiac injury had higher mortality rates compared with those without (51.2% vs 4.55%, $P < 0.001$). Complications such as acute respiratory syndrome distress, electrolyte alteration, and acute kidney injury were prevalent in patients with cardiac injury, suggesting how the cardiac involvement plays a detrimental effect in the prognosis of these patients[33]

A recently published review, composed of 26 studies including a total of 11,685 patients, estimated a lower prevalence of acute myocardial injury among SARS-CoV-2–infected patients, with around 20% showing evidence of myocardial injury (detected through the sample of troponin and/or creatine-kinase MB). In discussing the physiopathological mechanisms, the investigators also suggest a possible clinical role of cardiac biomarkers in the risk stratification of COVID-19.[34,35]

A systematic review published in 2021 estimated the rate of new cardiac injury between 7.2% and 77%, respectively, in live and dead SARS-CoV-2–infected cases, reiterating the concept that cardiac injury is associated to worse outcomes and higher rates of mortality, predominantly driven by development of shock and malignant arrythmias. In fact, about 46.3% of patients with cardiac injury required mechanical ventilation, 58.5% experienced acute respiratory distress syndrome, and 15.9% suffered from electrolyte disturbance. In addition, the levels of troponin I seemed to be inversely correlated with the days of survival.[36]

In a multicenter retrospective cohort study including 2736 patients, 36% were found to have elevated troponin concentration. Even small increases in troponin I levels (ranging from 0.03 to 0.09 ng/mL), found in the 16% of the entire cohort of patients, were significantly associated with the death of the patients (adjusted hazard ratio: 1.75; 95% confidence interval [CI]: 1.37–2.24; $P < .001$). Patients with evidence of more robust damage to the myocardium may experience more than a 3-fold increase in the risk of mortality. Patients with preexisting CVD are more likely to experience myocardial injury compared with those without.[37]

PRINCIPAL IMAGING FINDINGS IN PATIENTS WITH COVID-19 WITH MYOCARDIAL INJURY

The clinical presentation of myocardial injury in patients with COVID-19 is usually atypical and therefore hard to diagnose. The cause of the increase in troponin levels in patients with COVID-19 has not been clearly defined. Cardiac damage can arise in patients with no previous history of CVD and in the absence of chest pain. Diagnosing pathologies such as myocarditis in patients with COVID-19 and increased levels of troponin is quite challenging, given the scarcity of studies that correlate the evidence from imaging techniques such as cardiac MRI or invasive methods such as endomyocardial biopsy to the clinical and echocardiographic findings in these patients. In addition, the latency between the onset of symptoms and the evidence of myocardial injury (about 14 days) raises doubts as to whether myocyte damage can be considered only as a marker of advanced disease severity or if it directly implies a greater risk of COVID-19 mortality.[8,38–40] A recent study evaluating a total of 201 patients with COVID-19 with critical and noncritical clinical conditions and with myocardial injury, detected through an elevation of CK-MB and troponin I levels, reported 18.7% of cases showing evidence of echocardiographic abnormalities. The main abnormalities were right ventricular dilatation and dysfunction (prevalent in critical patients). The investigators were able to highlight the direct contribution of COVID-19 to the myocardial injury of these patients. In addition, 43.7% of patients had new changes at electrocardiography and 36.3% had signs of ST depression.[41]

Cardiac MRI (CMR) represents the hallmark of the morphologic definition and classification of myocardial tissue pathology, especially in patients with myocardial edema. In a systematic review by Ojha and colleagues including 199 patients from 34 studies, myocarditis was the most common diagnosis at cardiac MRI in patients with evidence of myocardial injury (40.2% of cases). Mapping abnormalities, edema, and late gadolinium enhancement (LGE) represented the most frequently detected myocardial findings.[42] In a prospective observational trial by Puntmann and colleagues including 100 recently recovered COVID-19 cases, abnormal findings at CMR were found in 78% of patients, of which 60% showed ongoing myocardial inflammation with an increased native T2 (in a minority of cases regional scar and pericardial enhancement were detected), regardless of preexisting conditions and COVID-19 severity, raising concerns on the long-term consequences of SARS-CoV-2.[43] Most of the patients experienced only mild forms of illness.[43]

The prevalence of cardiac damage at CMR was quite lower in another recent multicenter trial involving 148 cases of severe COVID-19 recruited from 6 different facilities and with laboratory evidence of troponin elevation. The trial evaluated patients after discharge through CMR. The CMR protocol included adenosine stress perfusion (where clinically appropriate) and was performed at a median of 68 days postdischarge. Twenty-six percent of CMRs showed evidence of a myocarditis-like scar, 22% of infarction or ischemia, and 6% characterized by combination of both. Most of the myocarditis-like lesions involved 3 or less segments and was not accompanied by left ventricular dysfunction, although 30% of these patients had active myocarditis. Stress perfusion revealed inducible ischemia in 26% of cases and myocardial infarction findings in 19%. These findings suggest how even after discharge the rate of cardiac injury remains high. About a quarter of all patients included in the trial experienced ischemic heart disease (in the absence of previous CVD history in two-thirds of cases).[44] The discrepancy in prevalence of cardiac abnormalities at CMR that emerges from the 2 previously cited studies can be explained by differences in the selection of study participants and in the definition of myocardial injury and inflammation using isolated or combined CMR parameters and, in addition, by the different latency periods between the acute phase of COVID-19 and the timing of CMR. Moreover, abnormal T1 sequences and LGE may overdiagnose myocardial inflammation if used alone. The studies did not investigate the possibility of underlying and silent pathologic cardiac conditions not directly related to COVID-19. Several limitations affected these studies, including the absence of a description of patients' symptoms and their correlation to imaging findings.[45] A recent literature review examining 277 patients with COVID-19 undergoing autopsy showed that the true prevalence of myocarditis was lower than 2%. Cardiovascular histopathologic findings potentially related to COVID-19 infections were found in the 47.8% of cases. The findings included myocardial microvascular thrombi, inflammation, or intraluminal megakaryocytes The investigators specified that the wide differences in histology reports found in the studies may be a marker of observer bias.[46] There are several ongoing studies with larger sample sizes, an accurate standard protocol of imaging assessment, and longer follow-up periods that aim to explore the mid- and long-term cardiac sequelae following COVID-19 and identify factors that could significantly affect the outcomes of these patients.

MYOCARDIAL INFARCTION TYPE 1, 2, AND 3

This paragraph explores the challenges in the management of the different types of MI and the possible overlap of acute pathologies (whether myocardial, pulmonary, or systemic) that further nuance the diagnosis.[47,48]

The largest study investigating COVID-19 and acute cardiovascular events is a Swedish study involving 86,742 patients diagnosed with COVID-19 and a matched population of controls (348,481 patients). The investigators calculated the incidence rate ratio (IRR) of acute MI following COVID-19. The IRR was calculated in 2 separate analyses: including the day of exposure to SARS-CoV-2 (day 0) and excluding day 0. Excluding day 0 from the analysis led to the estimation of the IRR of acute MI of 2.89 (95% CI 1.51–5.55) in the first week of infection and 2.53 (95% CI 1.29–4.94), and 1.60 (95% CI 0.84–3.04), respectively, in the second week and in the third and fourth weeks. The inclusion of day 0 in the analysis resulted in a significant increase in the IRR during the first week (IRR 8.44; 95% CI 5.45–13.08) followed by comparable rate ratios in the remaining weeks. The analysis that excludes the day of viral exposure ensures potential elimination of testing bias because there is a possibility of a higher likelihood of detecting even asymptomatic forms of SARS-COV-2 in patients who are admitted to the hospital for MI or ischemic stroke. On the other hand, the exclusion of the day of viral exposure may lead to an underestimation of the true risk of cardiovascular events.[49] These results seem to clash with the significant reduction in hospital admission rates for acute ischemic cardiovascular events (both acute coronary syndromes and ischemic strokes) that has been described during the initial phases of the pandemic.[50,51] A possible explanation of this discrepancy is that particularly during the first wave of the pandemic several patients experiencing ACS and acute ischemic stroke did not seek timely medical attention for fear of exposure to SARS-CoV-2 at the hospital or to respect measures of physical distancing. Another possible explanation is related to the clinical instability of patients with COVID-19 and the rapid deterioration of the conditions of patients with severe forms, preventing a complete diagnostic evaluation.[49,52]

There are also certain characteristics of patients hospitalized for STEMI and affected by COVID-19 that have been recently described in the literature and that raise concern among providers. Specifically, a study including a nationwide registry of 1010 consecutive patients treated within 42 specific STEMI care networks investigated the clinical, procedural, and in-hospital prognostic features of COVID-19 patients affected by STEMI. This population showed a significant increase in stent thrombosis (3.3% vs 0.8%, P = .020), cardiogenic shock (9.9% vs 3.8%, P = .007), and in-hospital mortality compared with non-COVID-19 STEMI patients (23.1% vs 5.7%, P < .0001).[53]

A single-center observational study of 115 consecutive patients with STEMI managed by primary percutaneous coronary intervention (PCI) showed a higher thrombus burden and higher rates of multivessel thrombosis (17.9% vs 0%, P = .003) and stent thrombosis (10.3% vs 1.2%, P = .04) in patients with COVID-19 compared with non-COVID patients. Although the thrombolysis in MI flow and thrombus grade were similar in the 2 groups, the modified thrombus grade after first device resulted higher in patients with COVID-STEMI (75% vs 31%; P = 1/4 0.0006). Of these cases of COVID-STEMI a high percentage (about 60% vs 9.2% P = .002) received a Gp IIb/IIIa and underwent thrombectomy (17.9% vs 1.3%) when compared with non-COVID patients. The patients in the COVID-19 group had higher proportions of hypertension, diabetes, dyslipidemia, and previous PCI. The myocardial blush grade (MBG) resulted significantly lower in the COVID-STEMI (MBG of 2–3 in 54% vs 93%, P < .0001); the postprocedural median left ventricular ejection fraction resulted lower in COVID-STEMI patients (42.5% vs 45.0%; P = .019) as well as higher peak plasma troponin levels. The higher thrombus burden found in the COVID-STEMI group may represent a requirement for a more aggressive antithrombotic therapy in selected cases, although the actual evidence supporting this conduct is still poor.[54]

Data investigating ACS and COVID-19 remain conflictual, and the association is still uncertain. A systematic review and meta-analysis including 50,123 patients from 10 studies revealed a non-statistically significant difference in admission rates of patients with STEMI during the pandemic compared with the previous year (IRR = 0.789, 95% CI 0.730–0.852 P = .01) and no increases in mortality for STEMI patients treated during the pandemic (odds ratio [OR] = 1.178, 95% CI 0.926–1.498, P = .01). What emerged from this review is that door-to-balloon time was significantly prolonged in STEMIs treated during the pandemic. Although these results harbor uncertainty regarding the impact of the pandemic on STEMI admission rates or mortality, they shed light on the organizational strain that facilities faced in the midst of the pandemic response.[55]

Diagnosis and management in patients with type 2 MI and COVID-19 are challenging, with repercussions on time to coronary angiographic evaluation. Inaccurate diagnosis of type 1 MI instead of type 2 and difficulties with differential diagnosis between MI and myocarditis might lead to an overestimation of acute MI. In a study by Stefanini and colleagues conducted on 28 patients with a diagnosis of STEMI that were promptly referred to the catheterization laboratory for urgent coronary angiography, 60.7% had a culprit lesion requiring urgent percutaneous treatment, whereas 39.3% did not show any signs of coronary obstructive lesion at angiography.[56]

Unfortunately the investigators did not investigate if the clinical presentation was attributable to a type 2 MI or to myocarditis or to SARS-CoV-2–related endothelial dysfunction. It is reasonable to hypothesize that a type 2 MI due to demand ischemia might be much more common in patients experiencing COVID-19. The condition of systemic inflammation triggered by viral infections, such as coronavirus and influenza virus,[57] may lead to oxygen supply–demand mismatch in the myocardium. It is also critical to highlight that it is clinically challenging to perform a correct differential diagnosis between non-STEMI ACS from other conditions that imply a form of myocardial injury such as hypoxemia, arrhythmias, sepsis, or myocarditis. To further complicate the matter, it is possible that these conditions may overlap, particularly in complex patients experiencing severe COVID-19. Sudden cardiac deaths or unexplained deaths have been reported in patients with SARS-CoV-2 infection and a previously diagnosed coronary artery disease. In this subset of

patients it is possible to speculate a type 3 MI as the cause of the demise.[58–60]

The Takotsubo syndrome (TTS) is another cardiomyopathy that may determine myocardial injury in patients with COVID-19. TTS consists in a transient acute myocardial dysfunction, often characterized by circumferential myocardial regional akinesia/hypokinesia, leading to clinical acute heart failure, and in some cases mimicking an acute MI. Although the definite physiopathology of TTS has not yet been totally clarified, it is known that the sympathetic stimulation (ie, catecholamine-induced microvascular impairment) driven by sudden stress represents a trigger, and other evidences suggest how ongoing inflammation, infections, and other clinical conditions such as respiratory failure may be involved in the etiology.[61]

A case series of 118 consecutive patients with COVID-19 undergoing transthoracic evaluation found ultrasound features of TTS in 4.2%. These patients also had higher level of plasmatic troponin compared with patients without TTS myocardial injury and high rates of in-hospital complications and mortality.[62] These findings are in line with the findings of other investigators who reported high rates of severe respiratory and cardiac insufficiency eventually leading to greater oxygen requirements, use of vasopressors, and cardiac ventricular support devices in patients with TTS myocardial injury associated with COVID-19.[63–65]

The available evidence on COVID-19 and myocardial injury highlights the necessity to perform an accurate evaluation of the troponin elevation (ie, of the myocardial injury), the patients' clinical features, and an appropriate risk stratification. Direct invasive testing should be reserved for patients with a high pretest probability of coronary artery disease (CAD), whereas computed tomography scan or CMR is the appropriate test for patients with an intermediate probability of CAD, in order to evaluate either epicardial arteries or coronary arteries and rule out myocarditis. Patients with a low risk of CAD should be referred to strict follow-up.

Patients with COVID-19 that in addition experience an STEMI or very high-risk NSTEMI should be referred to the catheterization laboratory within the timeframe suggested by the current guidelines. Fibrinolysis should be considered only in case of difficulties in patients' transfer to a hub center in order to perform timely PCIs.[66,67]

MULTISYSTEM INFLAMMATORY SYNDROME IN CHILDREN

Although COVID-19 usually represents a mild entity among children, with approximately 2% to 6% requiring intensive care, the infection should not be underestimated in the pediatric population.[68] A multisystem inflammatory syndrome (MIS-C) caused by SARS-CoV-2 has been reported among the pediatric population from several countries. MIS-C can lead to a large spectrum of symptoms that mimic a Kawasaki-like disease. Clinical manifestations range from persistent pyrexia to polymorphic rash, conjunctivitis, mucosal abnormalities, and myocardial involvement (including acute myocardial dysfunction, arrythmias, and acute pericarditis).[68]

Once again the cytokine storm plays a role in the pathogenesis of MIS-C. The condition of hyperinflammation can generate multiple consequences within the cardiac district. In severe cases there have been reports of coronary artery dilatation and aneurysm (8%–24% of patients), which may be due to the state of hyperinflammation with disruption of the arterial wall, as seen in Kawasaki disease (KD).[69]

Other clinical features described in children affected by MIS-C are acute myocardial dysfunction, hypotension requiring fluid resuscitation, and, in some cases, cardiogenic shock requiring cardiac inotropic support, mechanical ventilation, and extracorporeal membrane oxygenation.[69]

A key clinical difference between MIS-C and KD is represented by the fact that ventricular dysfunction and eventually shock are common presentations in MIS-C (50% of cases) and occur less frequently in children with KD (5%–10%).[69]

Recent evidence suggests that the administration of immunomodulatory drugs during the acute phase of the illness, such as intravenous immunoglobulins and steroids, may reverse the dysregulated inflammatory response yielding to recovery within days or a few weeks. Anticoagulation therapy is also suggested in the pediatric patients presenting with severe ventricular dysfunction and in case of evidence of giant coronary aneurysm.[69]

Although MIS-C is associated to low mortality, nothing is known of its mid- and long-term sequelae.

SUMMARY

Based on the current literature on myocardial injury during COVID-19, it is possible to conclude that this association is not uncommon. Myocardial injury can be considered as a concerning complication of SARS-CoV-2 infection, which can eventually lead to a large spectrum of myocardial pathologies (ie, myocarditis, myocardial infarction, Takotsubo syndrome) through the interaction between the virus and myocardial and endothelial cells, mediated by direct viral invasion or indirect mechanisms such as the downregulation of ACE2 receptor expression. Immune-mediated overresponse, cytokine storm, and activation of prothrombotic pathways are further mechanisms of myocardial damage that contribute to the various forms of myocardial injury that have been described.[22,23,70]

Although a trend of reduction in the number of hospital admissions for MI has been described, particularly during the first wave of pandemic, it is necessary to interpret these findings with caution and to consider the weight of other factors such as patient's reluctance to seek medical attention due to fear of in-hospital SARS-CoV-2 exposure or the strain on the organizational capacity of facilities in building the response to the pandemic.[49,52,71]

The direct impact of acute myocardial injury on the mortality of patients with COVID-19 has been described, whereas there is also evidence of long-term sequelae of myocardial injury (both inflammatory and ischemic) that are particularly concerning in older patients and in patients with cardiovascular comorbidities.[72]

There is therefore a pressing need to continue investigating these new and complex clinical entities in order to understand how to treat and manage these patients. It is possible to hypothesize the need for dedicated protocols that involve a strict cardiovascular follow-up through both clinical and sequential imaging evaluation, based on the patients' comorbidities and overall risk stratification.

CLINICS CARE POINTS

- Myocardial injury during COVID-19 can manifest through a large spectrum of pathologies (myocarditis, myocardial infarction, Takostubo Syndrome and MIS-C).

- Cardiac damage during SARS-CoV-2 infection can arise in patients with no previous hystory of heart disease or in the absence of symptoms and is therefore challenging to diagnose.

- There is evidence of long-term effects in patients affected by myocardial injury during SARS-CoV-2 infection, although the impact and reversibility of these sequelae is still not fully understood.

- Patients that experience myocardial injury during COVID-19 should undergo regular follow-up through clinical and imaging evaluation and dedicated protocols should be designed, based on their individual risk.

CONFLICT OF INTEREST

All the authors report no conflict of interest.

REFERENCES

1. Long B, Brady WJ, Koyfman A, et al. Cardiovascular complications in COVID-19. Am J Emerg Med 2020 Jul;38(7):1504–7.
2. Huang C, Wang Y, Li X, et al. Clinical features of patients infected with 2019 novel coronavirus in Wuhan, China. Lancet 2020;395:497–506.
3. Guan WJ, Ni ZY, Hu Y, et al. China medical treatment expert group for covid-19. Clinical characteristics of coronavirus disease 2019 in China. N Engl J Med 2020;382(18):1708–20.
4. Efros O, Barda N, Meisel E, et al. Myocardial injury in hospitalized patients with COVID-19 infection-Risk factors and outcomes. PLoS One 2021;16(2): e0247800.
5. Sheth AR, Grewal US, Patel HP, et al. Possible mechanisms responsible for acute coronary events in COVID-19. Med Hypotheses 2020;143:110125.
6. Puelles VG, Lütgehetmann M, Lindenmeyer MT, et al. Multiorgan and renal tropism of SARS-CoV-2. N Engl J Med 2020;383(6):590–2.
7. Gu ZC, Zhang C, Kong LC, et al. Incidence of myocardial injury in coronavirus disease 2019 (COVID-19): a pooled analysis of 7,679 patients from 53 studies. Cardiovasc Diagn Ther 2020;10(4):667–77.
8. Giustino G, Croft LB, Stefanini GG, et al. Characterization of myocardial injury in patients with COVID-19. J Am Coll Cardiol 2020;76(18):2043–55.
9. Oudit GY, Kassiri Z, Jiang C, et al. SARS-coronavirus modulation of myocardial ACE2 expression and inflammation in patients with SARS. Eur J Clin Invest 2009;39:618–25.
10. Babapoor-Farrokhran S, Gill D, Walker J, et al. Myocardial injury and COVID-19: possible mechanisms. Life Sci 2020;253:117723.
11. Laghlam D, Jozwiak M, Nguyen LS. Renin-angiotensin-aldosterone system and immunomodulation: a state-of-the-art review. Cells 2021;10(7):1767.
12. Hoffmann M, Kleine-Weber H, Schroeder S, et al. SARS-CoV-2 cell entry depends on ACE2 and TMPRSS2 and is blocked by a clinically proven protease inhibitor. Cell 2020;181(2):271–80. e8.
13. Li W, Moore MJ, Vasllieva N, et al. Angiotensin-converting enzyme 2 is a functional receptor for the SARS coronavirus. Nature 2003;426(6965):450–4.
14. Huang Y, Yang C, Xu XF, et al. Structural and functional properties of SARS-CoV-2 spike protein: potential antivirus drug development for COVID-19. Acta Pharmacol Sin 2020;41(9):1141–9.
15. Liu PP, Blet A, Smyth D, et al. The science underlying COVID-19: implications for the cardio- vascular system. Circulation 2020;142:68–78.
16. Sankrityayan H, Kale A, Sharma N, et al. Evidence for use or disuse of renin-angiotensin system modulators in patients having COVID-19 with an underlying cardiorenal disorder. J Cardiovasc Pharmacol Ther 2020;25(4):299–306.
17. Walls AC, Park YJ, Tortorici MA, et al. Structure, function, and antigenicity of the SARS-CoV-2 spike glycoprotein. Cell 2020;181(2):281–92.e6.
18. Kuba K, Imai Y, Penninger JM. Angiotensin-converting enzyme 2 in lung diseases. Curr Opin Pharmacol 2006;6(3):271–6.
19. Arentz M, Yim E, Klaff L, et al. Characteristics and outcomes of 21 critically ill patients with COVID-19 in Washington State. JAMA 2020;323:1612–4.
20. Liu Y, Yang Y, Zhang C, et al. Clinical and biochemical indexes from 2019-nCoV infected patients linked to viral loads and lung injury. Sci China Life Sci 2020;63:364–74.
21. Zhou F, Yu T, Du R, et al. Clinical course and risk factors for mortality of adult inpatients with COVID-19 in Wuhan, China: a retrospective cohort study. The Lancet 2020;395:1054–62.
22. Chen L, Li X, Chen M, et al. The ACE2 expression in human heart indicates new potential mechanism of heart injury among patients infected with SARS-CoV-2. Cardiovasc Res 2020;116(6):1097–100.
23. Mehta P, McAuley DF, Brown M, et al. HLH across Speciality Collaboration, UK. COVID-19: consider cytokine storm syndromes and immunosuppression. Lancet 2020;395(10229):1033–4.
24. Clerkin KJ, Fried JA, Raikhelkar J, et al. COVID-19 and cardiovascular disease. Circulation 2020; 141(20):1648–55.
25. Moccia F, Gerbino A, Lionetti V, et al. COVID-19-associated cardiovascular morbidity in older adults: a position paper from the Italian Society of Cardiovascular Researches. Geroscience 2020;42(4): 1021–49.
26. Tay MZ, Poh CM, Rénia L, et al. The trinity of COVID-19: immunity, inflammation and interven- tion. Nat Rev Immunol 2020;20:363–74.
27. Ramadan MS, Bertolino L, Marrazzo T, et al. The Monaldi Hospital Cardiovascular Infection Study Group. Cardiac complications during the active phase of COVID-19: review of the current evidence. Intern Emerg Med 2021;1–11.
28. Nencioni A, Trzeciak S, Shapiro NI. The microcirculation as a diagnostic and therapeutic target in sepsis. Intern Emerg Med 2009;4(5):413–8.
29. Xiong TY, Redwood S, Prendergast B, et al. Coronaviruses and the cardiovascular system: acute and long-term implications. Eur Heart J 2020;41(19): 1798–800.
30. Perrotta F, Corbi G, Mazzeo G, et al. COVID-19 and the elderly: insights into pathogenesis and clinical decision-making. Aging Clin Exp Res 2020;32(8): 1599–608.

31. Thygesen K, Alpert JS, Jaffe AS, et al. Executive group on behalf of the Joint European Society of Cardiology (ESC)/American College of Cardiology (ACC)/American heart association (AHA)/World heart Federation (WHF) Task Force for the Universal definition of myocardial infarction. Fourth universal definition of myocardial infarction (2018). J Am Coll Cardiol 2018;72(18):2231–64.

32. Bonow RO, Fonarow GC, O'Gara PT, et al. Association of coronavirus disease 2019 (COVID-19) with myocardial injury and mortality. JAMA Cardiol 2020;5(7):751–3.

33. Shi S, Qin M, Shen B, et al. Association of cardiac injury with mortality in hospitalized patients with COVID-19 in Wuhan, China [published online March 25, 2020]. JAMA Cardiol 2020;5(7):802–10.

34. Bavishi C, Bonow RO, Trivedi V, et al. Special article—acute myocardial injury in patients hospitalized with COVID-19 infection: a review. Prog Cardiovasc Dis 2020;63:682–9.

35. Nishiga M, Wang DW, Han Y, et al. COVID- 19 and cardiovascular disease: from basic mechanisms to clinical perspectives. Nat Rev Cardiol 2020;17: 543–58.

36. Moayed MS, Rahimi-Bashar F, Vahedian-Azimi A, et al. Cardiac injury in COVID-19: a systematic review. Adv Exp Med Biol 2021;1321:325–33.

37. Lala A, Johnson KW, Januzzi JL, et al. Prevalence and impact of myocardial injury in patients hospitalized with COVID-19 infection. J Am Coll Cardiol 2020;76:533–46.

38. Guo T, Fan Y, Chen M, et al. Cardiovascular implications of fatal outcomes of patients with coronavirus disease 2019 (COVID-19). JAMA Cardiol 2020;27:1–8.

39. Shi S, Qin M, Shen B, et al. Association of cardiac injury with mortality in hospitalized patients with COVID-19 in Wuhan, China. JAMA Cardiol 2020; 25:802–10.

40. Romero J, Alviz I, Parides M, et al. T-wave inversion as a manifestation of COVID-19 infection: a case series. J Interv Card Electrophysiol 2020;59(3):485–93.

41. Liaqat A, Ali-Khan RS, Asad M, et al. Evaluation of myocardial injury patterns and ST changes among critical and non-critical patients with coronavirus-19 disease. Sci Rep 2021;4828.

42. Ojha V, Verma M, Pandey NN, et al. Cardiac magnetic resonance imaging in coronavirus disease 2019 (COVID-19): a systematic review of cardiac magnetic resonance imaging findings in 199 patients. J Thorac Imaging 2021;36:73–83.

43. Puntmann VO, Carerj ML, Wieters I, et al. Outcomes of cardiovascular magnetic resonance imaging in patients recently recov- ered from coronavirus disease 2019 (COVID-19). JAMA Cardiol 2020;5: 1265–73.

44. Kotecha T, Knight DS, Razvi Y, et al. Patterns of myocardial injury in recovered troponin-positive COVID-19 patients assessed by cardiovascular magnetic resonance European Heart. Journal 2021;42(Issue 19):1866–78.

45. Friedrich MG, Cooper LT. What we (don't) know about myocardial injury after COVID-19. Eur Heart J 2021;42(Issue 19):1879–82.

46. Halushka MK, Vander Heide RS. Myocarditis is rare in COVID-19 autopsies: car- diovascular findings across 277 postmortem examinations. Cardiovasc Pathol 2021;50:107300.

47. Solomon MD, McNulty EJ, Rana JS, et al. The COVID-19 pandemic and the incidence of acute myocardial infarction. N Engl J Med 2020;383:691–9.

48. Tejada Meza H, Lambea Gil Á, Saldaña AS, et al. Impact of COVID-19 outbreak on ischemic stroke admissions and in-hospital mortality in North-West Spain. Int J Stroke 2020;15:755–62.

49. Katsoularis I, Fonseca-Rodriguez O, et al. Risk of acute myocardial infarction and ischaemic stroke following COVID-19 in Sweden: a self-controlled case series and matched cohort study Lancet 2021;398(10300):599–607.

50. Mafham MM, Spata E, Goldacre R, et al. COVID-19 pandemic and admission rates for and management of acute coronary syndromes in England. Lancet 2020;396:381–9.

51. D'Anna L, Brown M, Oishi S, et al. Impact of national lockdown on the hyperacute stroke care and rapid transient ischaemic attack outpatient service in a comprehensive tertiary stroke centre during the COVID-19 pandemic. Front Neurol 2021;12:627493.

52. Rudilosso S, Laredo C, Vera V, et al. Acute stroke care is at risk in the era of COVID-19: experience at a comprehensive stroke center in Barcelona. Stroke 2020;51:1991–5.

53. Rodriguez-Leor O, Cid Alvarez AB, Pérez de Prado A. In-hospital outcomes of COVID-19 ST-elevation myocardial infarction patients. EuroIntervention 2021;16:1426–33.

54. Choudry FA, Hamshere SM, Rathod KS, et al. High thrombus burden in patients with COVID-19 presenting with ST-Segment elevation myocardial infarction. J Am Coll Cardiol 2020;76(10):1168–76.

55. Rattka M, Dreyhaupt J, Winsauer C, et al. Effect of the COVID- 19 pandemic on mortality of patients with STEMI: a systematic review and meta-analysis. Heart 2020;107:482–7.

56. Stefanini GG, Montorfano M, Trabattoni D, et al. ST-elevation myocardial infarction in patients with COVID-19: clinical and angiographic outcomes. Circulation 2020;141:2113–6.

57. Smeeth L, Thomas SL, Hall AJ, et al. Risk of myocardial infarction and stroke after acute infection or vaccination. N Engl J Med 2004;351:2611–8.

58. Ebinger JE, Shah PK. Declining admissions for acute cardiovascular illness: the Covid-19 paradox. J Am Coll Cardiol 2020;76:289–91.

59. Metzler B, Siostrzonek P, Binder RK, et al. Decline of acute coronary syn- drome admissions in Austria since the outbreak of COVID-19: the pandemic response causes cardiac collateral damage. Eur Heart J 2020;41:1852–3.

60. De Rosa S, Spaccarotella C, Basso C, et al. Reduction of hospitalizations for myocardial infarction in Italy in the COVID-19 era. Eur Heart J 2020;41: 2083–8.

61. Medina de Chazal H, Del Buono MG, Keyser-Marcus L, et al. Stress cardiomyopathy diagnosis and treatment: JACC state-of-the-art review. J Am Coll Cardiol 2018;72:1955–71.

62. Giustino G, Croft LB, Oates CP, et al. Takotsubo cardiomyopathy in males with Covid-19. J Am Coll Cardiol 2020;76:628–9.

63. Roca E, Lombardi C, Campana M, et al. Takotsubo syndrome associated with COVID-19. Eur J Case Rep Intern Med 2020;7:001665.

64. Park JH, Moon JY, Sohn KM, et al. Two fatal cases of stress-induced cardiomyopathy in COVID-19 patients. J Cardio- Vasc Imaging 2020;28:300–3.

65. Nguyen D, Nguyen T, De Bels D, et al. A case of Takotsubo cardiomyopathy with COVID 19. Eur Heart J Cardiovasc Imaging 2020;21:1052.

66. Cameli M, Pastore MC. Giulia Elena Mandoli et al COVID-19 and Acute Coronary Syndromes: current Data and Future Implications. Front Cardiovasc Med 2021;7:593496.

67. Impact of COVID-19 pandemic on mechanical reperfusion for patients with STEMI. De Luca G, Verdoia M, Cerchek M et al. Am Coll Cardiol 2020; 76(20):2321–30.

68. Sperotto F, Friedman K, Son MB, et al. Cardiac manifestations in SARS-CoV-2-associated multisystem inflammatory syndrome in children: a comprehensive review and proposed clinical approach. Eur J Pediatr 2021;180(2):307–22.

69. Alsaied T, Tremoulet AH, Burns JC, et al. Review of cardiac involvement in multisystem inflammatory syndrome in children. Circulation 2021;143(1): 78–88.

70. Della Rocca DG, Magnocavallo M, Lavalle C, et al. Evidence of systemic endothelial injury and microthrombosis in hospitalized COVID-19 patients at different stages of the disease. J Thromb Thrombolysis 2021;51(3):571–6.

71. Versaci F, Scappaticci M, Calcagno S, et al. ST-elevation myocardial infarction in the COVID-19 era. Minerva Cardiol Angiol 2021;69(1):6–8.

72. De Luca G, Cercek M, Jensen LO, et al. Impact of COVID-19 pandemic and diabetes on mechanical reperfusion in patients with STEMI: insights from the ISACS STEMI COVID 19 Registry. Cardiovasc Diabetol 2020;19(1):215.

Clinical Features and Management of COVID-19– Associated Hypercoagulability

Gianluca Massaro, MD[a], Dalgisio Lecis, MD[a], Eugenio Martuscelli, MD[a,b],
Gaetano Chiricolo, MD[a,b],*, Giuseppe Massimo Sangiorgi, MD[a,b]

KEYWORDS

- COVID-19 coagulopathy • Hypercoagulability • Venous thromboembolism • Arterial thrombosis
- Antithrombotic therapy

KEY POINTS

- COVID-19 is associated with blood coagulation changes leading to a prothrombotic state.
- Thrombotic complications affect more the venous than the arterial district.
- The incidence of thrombosis increases in more severe forms of the disease and is associated with high mortality.
- Management of hypercoagulability in COVID-19 is based on preventive measures in patients at risk or the treatment of manifest thrombotic complications.
- Anticoagulation is the most widely used therapy for the prevention and treatment of thrombosis associated with SARS-CoV-2 infection. Numerous trials are ongoing to define the best therapeutic strategy in the different clinical presentations of the disease.

INTRODUCTION

Coronavirus disease 2019 (COVID-19) is a viral illness caused by the severe acute respiratory syndrome coronavirus 2 (SARS-CoV-2). COVID-19 carries several important cardiovascular implications.[1,2] Since this pandemic disease broke out, it has been observed an increasing occurrence of thromboembolic events in patients without a history of cardiovascular disease.[3] The progressive acquisition of knowledge on the pathogenetic effects of SARS-CoV-2 infection has found a prominent role of the venous and arterial vascular system in the disease. Accumulated evidence has shown that coagulopathy is frequently observed in COVID-19 patients, especially in those with critical illness.[4] Han and colleagues[5] reported increased D-dimer values and fibrin/fibrinogen degradation products and reduced prothrombin time (PT)-activity in patients with COVID-19. The increase in D-dimer is particularly marked in severe patients and can be used in patient triaging and disease monitoring. SARS-CoV-2 infection in severe forms triggers a vicious cycle that includes hypercoagulability, endothelial cell activation, and massive release of inflammatory mediators[6] (Fig. 1). All this leads to an increased incidence of pulmonary and systemic thrombotic phenomena. A large series of autopsies documented an incidence of venous thromboembolism (VTE) of 42.5% and pulmonary embolism (PE) of 21%.[7] Among the most feared systemic complications of SARS-CoV-2 infection is disseminated intravascular coagulation (DIC), primarily characterized by thrombotic phenomena, with a lower incidence of bleeding and thrombocytopenia than other viral infections. Autopsies also revealed thrombotic microangiopathy observed in the lungs, termed

G. Massaro and D. Lecis contributed equally to the article conception and writing.
a Division of Cardiology, "Tor Vergata" University Hospital, v.le Oxford 81, Rome 00133, Italy; b Department of Biomedicine and Prevention, "Tor Vergata" University of Rome, Rome 00133, Italy
* Corresponding author. Division of Cardiology, "Tor Vergata" University Hospital, v.le Oxford 81, Rome 00133, Italy.
E-mail address: nucciochiricolo@gmail.com

Card Electrophysiol Clin 14 (2022) 41–52
https://doi.org/10.1016/j.ccep.2021.10.005

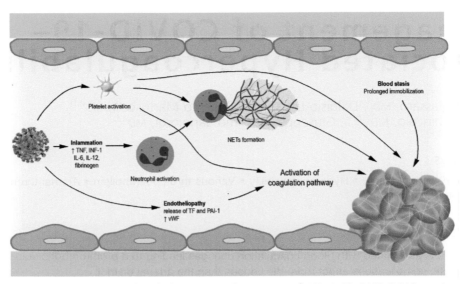

Fig. 1. Major mechanisms associated with the procoagulative state of COVID-19. SARS-CoV-2 exerts multiple effects systemically. Activation of the inflammatory response results in the recruitment of immune cells, including neutrophils. The virus can lead to a pathologic hyperactivation of platelets and endothelial damage that triggers the coagulation pathway.[17] Some evidence points to a role of activated platelets in stimulating NETosis. NETs contribute to the onset of thrombotic phenomena. All this is favored by blood stasis, due to prolonged immobilization typical of the most severe forms of the disease.[87] IL-6, interleukin-6; IL-12, interleukin-12; INF-1, interferon-1; NET, neutrophil extracellular trap; PAI-1, plasminogen activator inhibitor-1; TNF, tumor necrosis factor; TF, tissue factor; vWF, Von-Willebrand factor.

"pulmonary intravascular coagulopathy".[7] In severe COVID-19, the "cytokine storm" is associated with abnormal coagulation parameters. It has been noticed that, in COVID-19 patients, higher interleukin (IL)-6 blood levels are directly related to fibrinogen levels predisposing to a hypercoagulable state and thromboembolic events.[8] COVID-19–associated hypercoagulability can essentially be grouped into two main clinical manifestations: venous thrombotic events and arterial thrombotic events (ATEs) **(Fig. 2)**.

PATHOPHYSIOLOGY OF HYPERCOAGULABILITY

A major cause of morbidity and mortality in COVID-19 patients is thromboinflammation (the coordinated activation of thrombosis and inflammation). Laboratory tests revealed, in a great percentage of patients hospitalized with COVID-19, the evidence of a coagulopathy resembling DIC with marked elevated levels of D-dimers in the plasma, a mild prolongation of the PT, and borderline thrombocytopenia.[9] The postmortem examinations of COVID-19 patients showed extensive endothelial injury and diffuse microthrombosis.[10–12] However, the etiology of COVID-19–associated coagulopathy is still controversial and is

likely to be heterogeneous, involving many different cell types. Indeed, observational studies and case series showed that not all the COVID-19 patients admitted to the ICU fulfilled the ISTH criteria for DIC (elevation of D-dimer levels, moderate-to-severe thrombocytopenia, prolongation of PT time, and decreased fibrinogen levels). Goshua and colleagues observed that, in a cohort of critically ill patients with COVID-19, the platelet counts were typically normal or mildly elevated and fibrinogen levels were markedly increased: findings that are inconsistent with coagulopathy of consumption such as DIC.[13] The global interpretation from these diverse reports is that although COVID-19–associated coagulopathy has some shared pathophysiological features with DIC, the coagulopathy observed in patients with COVID-19 can be considered as a distinct entity. In COVID-19, the variable state of hypercoagulability depends both on the type of cell involvement (eg, endothelial cells, platelets, leukocytes) and the time of sample collection during the disease process. In patients with severe COVID-19, elevated levels of inflammatory markers (such as C-reactive protein, ferritin, erythrocyte sedimentation rate, and cytokines, including IL-1β, IL-6, and TNF) lead to a hyperinflammatory response known as "cytokine storm," which is

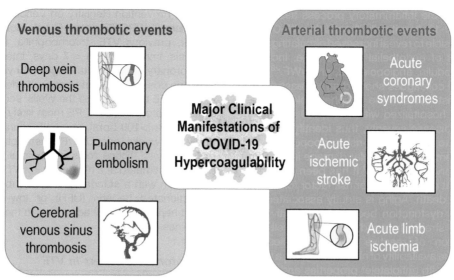

Fig. 2. Major thrombotic complications associated with COVID-19. Thromboses affect both arterial and venous districts. The latter are more frequent.

associated with poor outcomes. Jose and colleagues showed the correlation between elevated circulating levels of inflammatory cytokines and abnormal coagulation parameters.[14] The IL-6 levels have been shown to correlate directly with fibrinogen levels in patients with COVID-19,[8] as well as the levels of prothrombotic acute phase reactants (fibrinogen, vWF, and factor VIII) are increased in patients with COVID-19 compared with healthy individuals.[15,16] In a recent review, Gu and colleagues[17] identified platelets and endothelial cells as the two main cell types whose dysfunction contributes to the inflammation and coagulopathy associated with COVID-19, leading to thrombosis and eventually death. In the context of cardiovascular risk factors (diabetes mellitus, obesity, aging, and smoking), the mechanism of thrombocytopathy and endotheliopathy has been well represented. These findings are in line with the evidence that COVID-19 patients with cardiovascular risk factors have a high incidence of vascular complications (such as VTE, arterial thrombosis, and thrombotic microangiopathy), which contribute to the high mortality.[18–20]

Thrombocytopathy and Endotheliopathy in COVID-19

Contrary to what was thought in the past regarding their limited functions, platelets interact with many other cell types, including circulating blood cells and endothelial cells, either directly or through the release of signaling molecules, thus functioning as a blood component that bridges the immune system (through interactions with various leukocytes) and thrombosis (via platelet activation and release of hemostatic and inflammatory mediators).[21] Manne and colleagues demonstrated that platelets are hyperactivated in patients with COVID-19.[22] Activated platelets express on their surface some molecules involved in the stimulation of the immune system (such as P-selectin and CD40 L). Moreover, activated platelets can release α-granules, complement C3, and various cytokines (CCL2, IL-1β, IL-7, and IL-8), thus triggering the immune system activation camp.[23,24] Another cause of platelets hyperactivation is hypoxia,[25] a condition widely documented in COVID-19 patients who develop mild to severe hypoxia with peripheral blood oxygen desaturation. In addition, platelets dysfunction could be associated with a direct viral infection. ACE2, the cell-entry receptor for SARS-CoV-2, is expressed in the respiratory epithelium and endothelial cells,[26] but SARS-CoV-2 RNA traces were detected in platelet.[22] Other potential methods of SARS-CoV-2 entry into platelets independent of ACE2 are emerging.[27] At last, a potential mechanism for platelet hyperactivation and thrombocytopenia consists in the formation of immune complexes similar to that seen in heparin-induced thrombocytopenia (HIT) with the consequence of an increased platelet clearance.[28]

Endotheliopathy is a critical feature of severe COVID-19 across multiple studies. The endothelial damage and microvascular thrombosis are the results of both the direct viral infection of endothelial cells by SARS-CoV-2 and the endothelial cell response to the inflammatory process associated with COVID-19. In critically ill patients with COVID-19, it is possible to reveal increased circulating levels of markers of endothelial cell damage, including thrombomodulin, angiopoietin 2, and vWF.[29] Della Rocca and colleagues showed an increased number of schistocytes in the peripheral blood smear of patients hospitalized with COVID-19 at different stages of disease severity, thus identifying a new biomarker to reveal a high-risk subpopulation with latent systemic microvascular damage irrespective of respiratory symptoms.[30] It has been well documented that age is the major risk factor for COVID-19–related death. Aging is strictly associated with endothelial dysfunction because of oxidative and nitrosative stress. In aged endothelial cells, the accumulation of reactive oxygen species can decrease the availability of nitric oxide (NO), a potent vasodilator with antiplatelet properties and cardioprotective effects.[31] One of the most important functions of the vascular endothelium is to maintain a balance between proinflammatory and anti-inflammatory factors. In the elderly, the simultaneous invasion of the endothelium by SARS-CoV-2 via the angiotensin-converting enzyme 2 (ACE2) receptor can exacerbate endothelial dysfunction and damage, further promoting vascular inflammation and thrombosis.

VENOUS THROMBOTIC EVENTS IN COVID-19

A high incidence of thrombotic events, particularly deep vein thrombosis (DVT) and PE, has been documented in COVID-19 patients. As described in many studies, elevated D-dimer level is a common finding in COVID-19 patients. Anyway, high D-dimer levels meet low specificity in the absence of overt VTE clinical manifestations. Then, it is essential to recognize some "red flags" that can increase VTE suspicion in COVID-19 patients. The occurrence of typical DVT symptoms (asymmetric limb pain or edema), the increasing supplemental oxygen requirement, and hemodynamic instability in the setting of imaging findings inconsistent with worsening COVID-19 pneumonia or the onset of acute unexplained right ventricular dysfunction can be considered clinical manifestations of VTE.[32] Several scoring risk systems have been developed to help the clinician in the identification of VTE (**Table 1**). The most used are the Padua prediction score (including factors such as previous VTE, active cancer, reduced mobility, known thrombophilic condition, recent trauma or surgery, age ≥ 70 years, respiratory/cardiac failure, acute myocardial infarction/stroke, acute infection, obesity, and ongoing hormonal treatment; <4: low risk of VTE; ≥4: high risk of VTE), the International

Medical Prevention Registry on Venous Thromboembolism (IMPROVE) score (7 risk factors: active cancer, previous VTE, thrombophilia, lower limb paralysis, immobilization < 7 days, intensive care unit/coronary care unit stay, age > 60 years; more than one positive factor increases the risk of symptomatic VTE to 7.2%), and the Wells' score (clinical signs/symptoms of DVT, PE most likely diagnosis, tachycardia [>100 bpm], immobilization/surgery in previous 4 weeks, prior DVT/PE, hemoptysis, active malignancy).[33] These tools are helpful to identify patients estimated at a higher risk for VTE and start prevention with a standard dose of subcutaneous unfractionated heparin (UFH) or low-molecular-weight heparin (LMWH) according to the published guidelines.

Laboratory Parameters in VTE

The most consistent hemostatic abnormalities with COVID-19 include, as mentioned earlier, increased D-dimer levels.[34] A prospective study comparing coagulation parameter disorders among patients with COVID-19 and healthy controls suggested that the D-dimer levels (10.36 vs 0.26 ng/L; $P < .001$), fibrin/fibrinogen degradation products (33.83 vs 1.55 mg/L; $P < .001$), and fibrinogen (5.02 vs 2.90 g/L; $P < .001$), in all SARS-CoV-2 cases, were substantially higher than those in healthy controls. Moreover, these biomarkers, especially D-dimer and fibrinogen degradation products, were higher in patients with severe SARS-CoV-2 infection than those with mild disease.[5] Another common finding is mild thrombocytopenia. A meta-analysis showed that patients with severe disease were found to have a significantly lower platelet count (mean difference: -31×10^9/L; 95% confidence interval [CI], -35 to -29×10^9/L), and thrombocytopenia was associated with a 5-fold higher odds of having the severe disease (odds ratio: 5.13; 95% CI, 1.81–14.58).[35] Other hemostatic abnormalities variably associated with COVID-19 severity are the prolongation of the PT, international normalized ratio (INR),[13,14] and thrombin time.[36] A trend toward shortened activated partial thromboplastin time (aPTT) is variably associated with the disease severity.[37,38] Tang and colleagues[39] assessed 183 patients with COVID-19, 21 (11.5%) of whom died. The patients who died showed increased levels of D-dimer and fibrin degradation products (w3.5- and w1.9-fold, respectively) and PT prolongation (by 14%) ($P < .001$) when compared with survivors. Among the patients who died, 71% fulfilled the International Society on Thrombosis and Haemostasis (ISTH) criteria[40] for DIC, compared with only 0.6% among survivors. Taken all together, these

Table 1
Scoring systems commonly used for the assessment of the risk of venous thromboembolism and pulmonary embolism.

Items	Score
Padua Risk Score	
Active cancer (metastases and/or chemoradiotherapy in the previous 6 mo)	3
Previous VTE (with the exclusion of superficial vein thrombosis)	3
Bedrest for $\geq$ 3 d	3
Thrombophilia	3
Recent ($\leq$1 mo) trauma and/or surgery	2
Elderly age ($\geq$70 y)	1
Heart and/or respiratory failure	1
Acute myocardial infarction or ischemic stroke	1
Acute infection and/or rheumatologic disorder	1
Obesity (BMI $\geq$ 30 kg/m^2)	1
Ongoing hormonal treatment	1
High risk of VTE: $\geq$ 4 points	
IMPROVE score	
Previous VTE	3
Known thrombophilia	2
Current lower limb paralysis or paresis	2
History of cancer	2
ICU/CCU stay	1
Complete immobilization $\geq$ 1 d	1
Age $\geq$ 60 y	1
High-risk indication for prophylaxis if score $\geq$ 3	
Well's score	
Clinical signs/symptoms of DVT	3
PE is most likely diagnosis	3
Tachycardia (>100 bpm)	1.5
Immobilization/surgery in previous 4 wk	1.5
Prior DVT/PE	1.5
Hemoptysis	1
Active malignancy (trt w/in 6 mo)	1
Total score > 4: PE likely Total score < 4: PE unlikely	

Abbreviations: BMI, body mass index; CCU, cardiac care unit; DVT, deep venous thrombosis; ICU, intensive care unit; PE, pulmonary embolism; VTE, venous thromboembolism.

hemostatic abnormalities indicate some forms of coagulopathy that may predispose to thrombotic events. However, the underlying mechanism leading to the clinical manifestations of VTE is still unknown.

Nevertheless, it is uncertain whether these hemostatic changes are a specific effect of SARS-CoV-2 infection or are a consequence of the cytokine storm that precipitates the onset of systemic inflammatory response syndrome (SIRS) as documented in other severe viral diseases.[41,42] A recent study reported 3 cases with severe COVID-19 and cerebral infarction, with one associated with bilateral limb ischemia, in the setting of elevated antiphospholipid antibodies.[43] The presence of antiphospholipid antibodies (eg, anti-cardiolipin IgA, anti–β2-glycoprotein I IgA, and IgG) has been described in the serum of COVID-19 patients. This finding may contribute to an increased risk of both venous and arterial thrombosis.[44,45] However, some studies have highlighted that in setting a high degree of inflammation, like in SIRS, and an increased level of inflammatory markers, those antibodies can be falsely positive.[46] Whether antiphospholipid antibodies play a significant role in the pathophysiology of thrombosis associated with COVID-19 requires further investigation.

Imaging for VTE

To yield a definitive diagnosis of VTE, imaging studies can be helpful. The American Heart Association guidelines on managing massive and submassive PE recommend performing computed tomography pulmonary angiography (CTPA) in all patients with intermediate or high pretest probability or a positive D-dimer.[47] Referring to COVID-19, some studies have shown the usefulness of compression ultrasonography and CTPA in this setting of patients.[48,49] An Italian study showed that 16 (36%) of 44 consecutive symptomatic patients had VTE on imaging, and 10 (33%) of 30 patients had a PE at CTPA. Half of the thromboembolic events were diagnosed within 24 h of hospital admission, highlighting the significance of early diagnosis and treatment in patients with COVID-19.[50] The decision to perform an imaging study for diagnosing DVT should be based on clinical judgment. The feasibility of these imaging modalities (mainly ultrasound imaging) in COVID-19 is a matter of concern because of the prolonged health care assistants' exposition time. Therefore, the role of bedside point-of-care ultrasound is essential in aiding diagnosis, reducing the exposition time. In a recent multicenter study, a 100% sensitivity and a 95.8%

specificity have been showing resorting to point-of-care ultrasound for the diagnosis of DVT.[51] At last, in patients with high clinical suspicion of PE, a bedside cardiac ultrasound also assists with the diagnosis by rapid assessment of right ventricular size and function.

ATEs IN COVID-19

The relationship between viral respiratory infections and arterial thrombosis, especially acute coronary syndrome (ACS), is clearly described[52] Cases of ACS have been previously described with influenza or other viral illness. They have been attributed to a combination of SIRS as well as localized vascular or plaque inflammation.[53] During the COVID-19 pandemics, small series of patients with coronary, cerebrovascular, and peripheral ATEs have also been reported, but their true incidence and consequences are not well described. In a series of 18 patients with COVID-19 and ST-segment elevation, in more than 50% of them, the origin was considered to be noncoronary.[54] Acute limb ischemia has been reported in 2 young COVID-19 patients with occlusion of major arteries of the upper and lower limbs.[55] In the systematic review and meta-summary of Tan and colleagues, it has been reported that the incidence of acute ischemic stroke in COVID-19 patients ranges from 0.9% to 2.7%. From this meta-summary, it has been observed that acute ischemic stroke severity in COVID-19 patients is typically at least moderate (NIHSS score 19 ± 8), with a high prevalence (40.9%) of large vessel occlusion. Notably, a significant number of cases tested positive for antiphospholipid antibodies. Although it is reported that antiphospholipid antibodies are commonly found in COVID-19 infections, the true prevalence of antiphospholipid-antibody positivity in the general population is not known. It has also been detected in healthy individuals. Hence, the significance of antiphospholipid antibodies in the pathogenesis of acute ischemic stroke in COVID-19 patients remains uncertain. It may be worthwhile for future studies to repeat and trend these serologic markers after the acute thrombotic setting.

At last, the mortality rate of COVID-19 patients experiencing acute ischemic stroke has been reported high (38.0%).[56] Recently, Cantador and colleagues[57] observed the 1% incidence of systemic ATEs in a large cohort of 1419 COVID-19 patients, with a death rate of 28.6%. In this study, the incidence of thrombotic events, at least for cerebrovascular, seems to be higher than expected with very serious consequences. A meta-analysis conducted by Lippi and colleagues showed that cTnI concentration is only marginally increased in all patients with SARS-CoV-2 infection, whereby values exceeding the 99th percentile in the upper reference limit can only be observed in 8% to 12% of positive cases. Furthermore, higher troponin levels are associated with severe COVID-19.[58] Hence, it is reasonable to hypothesize that initial measurement of cardiac damage biomarkers immediately after hospitalization for SARS-CoV-2 infection, and longitudinal monitoring during the hospital stay may help identify a subset of patients with possible cardiac injury and thereby predict the progression of COVID-19 toward a worse clinical picture.[59] However, not all such events are due to thrombotic ACS. These data, taken all together, suggest that, although COVID-19 may favor the occurrence of thrombotic events, the destabilization and thrombosis of atherosclerotic plaques do not seem to be a frequent mechanism that warrants the need for specific systematic preventive measures. Nevertheless, a high level of suspicion and clinical surveillance should undoubtedly be maintained.

MANAGEMENT OF COVID-19–ASSOCIATED HYPERCOAGULABILITY

Coagulopathy associated with SARS-CoV-2 infection has peculiar characteristics compared with that associated with conventional sepsis, as evidenced by the difference in coagulation parameters described earlier. This is confirmed by the evidence of reduced mortality in patients with COVID-19 and elevated D-dimer undergoing anticoagulation than non–COVID-19 patients.[60]

COVID-19 disease is associated with a higher incidence of thrombotic than hemorrhagic complications, which is the rationale for pharmacologic schemes targeting the coagulation pathway.

In the early stages of the pandemic, the absence of randomized clinical trials (RCTs) forced physicians to take an empirical approach to the use of anticoagulant regimens. Early evidence of different clinical pictures and numerous variables characterizing COVID-19 disease led to the realization that the "one-size-fits-all" strategy was not feasible.

To date, more than 75 RCT testing anticoagulant regimens in different clinical settings have been designed.[61] The choice of drug and dosage in RCTs depends on the expected rate of thrombotic events in the study population: the use of prophylactic or intermediate doses has been preferred in trials of patients with mild COVID-19, whereas patients with critical illness or requiring intensive care have been treated with higher-dose regimens.

Given the higher incidence of thrombosis in venous versus arterial districts,[48,62] clinical trials have tested more pharmacologic regimens to prevent and treat VTE. The use of such strategies in different types of patients will be discussed in the following section.

Pharmacologic Approaches

The main approaches used in RCTs for the prevention and treatment of thrombotic complications of COVID-19 include UFH, LMWH, fondaparinux, direct oral anticoagulants (DOACs), antiplatelet drugs, direct parenteral thrombin inhibitors, fibrinolytic agents, and drugs less commonly used in clinical practice such as dociparstat, dipyridamole, and nafamostat. The most significant evidence is with heparins and antiplatelet drugs.

Data on head-to-head comparisons between different drugs are lacking, so the choice is often driven by practical considerations.

Their wide use, mainly in the hospital setting, has made heparins the most studied anticoagulant drugs to treat COVID-19 coagulopathy. In addition to its anticoagulant effect, heparin also has anti-inflammatory properties and protective effects on the endothelium.[63]

In prophylactic anticoagulation, once-daily LMWH is preferred over twice-daily subcutaneous UFH administration to reduce health care worker exposure. Therapeutic anticoagulation with UHF has the advantage that it can be temporarily discontinued and shows utility, especially in patients who are candidates for invasive procedures. However, frequent blood draws to check that aPTT is in the therapeutic range favor LMWH for the reasons already stated.

The antiviral and anti-inflammatory effects of heparin provide the rationale for the use of nebulized forms of UFH. Three trials are ongoing to test the efficacy and safety of this formulation compared to standard-of-care (INHALE-HEP and PACTR2020076032743) or prophylactic LMWH (NEBU-HEPA)

Direct anticoagulants represent an unquestionable advantage, especially in outpatients, to reduce the continuous recourse to INR assessment. However, their intrahospital use is limited by numerous interactions with other medications that are used to treat COVID-19 disease and the inability to use them in patients under orotracheal intubation or with dysphagia.

The use of antiplatelet drugs in the prophylaxis of thrombotic complications in patients with COVID-19 disease has been evaluated in both mild and severe forms of the disease. However,

unlike heparins, antiplatelet drugs have not demonstrated effects on "endotheliopathy."[17]

Prevention of VTE in Patients with Mild COVID-19

Patients with mild COVID-19 generally do not require hospitalization and should maintain home isolation. There are several ongoing clinical trials on the use of LMWH,[61] DOAC, or aspirin in these patients. The only clinical trial published to date tested the use of sulodexide in the early stages of the disease in 243 patients in preventing hospitalizations and the use of oxygen therapy. The treatment arm showed a reduction in hospitalizations (relative risk: 0.60; 95% CI, 0.37–0.96; $P = .03$) and in the need for oxygen support (relative risk: 0.71; 95% CI, 0.50–1.00; $P = .05$) compared with placebo, with no significant difference in mortality.

Current recommendations do not indicate antithrombotic prophylaxis in all patients. However, in subjects at high risk of VTE (immobility, procoagulative status, previous VTE), antithrombotic prophylaxis should be considered, also taking into account the risk of bleeding.

Prevention and Treatment of VTE in Hospitalized Patients

When the pandemic began its spread in Europe, in China, Tang and colleagues[64] demonstrated that, in patients hospitalized for COVID-19 and with high D-dimer or high sepsis-induced coagulopathy (SIC) score, 28-day mortality was lower among those receiving anticoagulation than among those not receiving it. Most of the treated patients had received LMWH at prophylactic doses. Therefore, the international societies agreed that prophylactic dose LMWH should be considered in all patients (including noncritically ill) who require hospital admission for COVID-19 infection in the absence of any contraindications.[65]

Anticoagulant dosing for the prevention of VTE is not well defined. Some clinicians use a therapeutic-dose anticoagulant regimen in the prevention of thrombotic complications in all hospitalized patients, whereas others reserve it for patients at high thrombotic risk, based on D-dimer or SIC score values. As already discussed, some evidence shows that SARS-CoV-2 disease has distinctive features compared with other forms of sepsis. Hadid and colleagues[66] have proposed a specific score for COVID-19 called CIC (COVID-19–induced coagulopathy) score, which adds the D-dimer value to the previous SIC score. Although not yet validated, this score can be helpful to estimate the risk of thrombotic complications and start more intensive anticoagulation in patients with severe disease.

An observational study in the United States showed a better outcome in hospitalized patients treated with treatment-dose of anticoagulants than in those treated with prophylactic-dose.[67] HESACOVID, a randomized phase 2 clinical trial, showed improved gas exchange and reduced need for mechanical ventilation in patients with severe COVID-19 receiving therapeutic enoxaparin compared with the group receiving prophylactic anticoagulation.[68]

Numerous clinical trials are ongoing to evaluate the use of different anticoagulant regimens in patients with severe disease. The design of the trials involves the use of more intense anticoagulation. In some studies, the administration of fibrinolytic agents is tested in patients with very severe forms, despite the rather limited sample size.

A complication observed in patients with severe forms of COVID-19 is DIC. Traditionally, DIC is characterized by thrombotic and hemorrhagic complications, whereas in the specific setting of SARS-CoV-2 disease, the former is more frequent than the latter. In patients with COVID-19 and DIC, prophylactic anticoagulation should be administered in the absence of overt bleeding. There is a tendency to recommend a less intense anticoagulation regimen in these patients; however, the individual risk of VTE and significant bleeding must be weighed.

Prevention of VTE in Postdischarge Patients

Some trials in acutely ill medical patients have shown that the extension of anticoagulation therapy after discharge is associated with reducing thromboembolic events at the cost of increased bleeding.[69] Given the particular tendency to hypercoagulability of patients with COVID-19, some trials evaluate the use of different pharmacologic regimens, including DOACs.[70,71]

Treatment of Arterial Thromboembolic Complications

Arterial complications of SARS-CoV-2 infection have received less attention because of their lower incidence compared with their venous counterparts.[48,62] A report from the New York City area shows that 57% of arterial thromboses, in patients with COVID-19 (upper- and lower limb ischemia, bowel ischemia, and cerebral ischemia), were treated with systemic anticoagulant therapy alone, 6% with administration of systemic tissue-plasminogen activator, 27% with revascularization, and 10% with amputation.[72]

Patients with acute coronary thrombosis and concomitant SARS-CoV-2 infection have a higher thrombotic burden and a worse prognosis.[73] Hospital admissions for ST-segment elevation myocardial infarction (STEMI) were reduced during the pandemic, with a more extended treatment delay and hospitalization.[74] The treatment of patients with STEMI and established or suspected COVID-19 raised essential questions. The proposal to increase thrombolysis to protect health care workers[75] was not adopted by the European Association of Percutaneous Cardiovascular Interventions (EAPCI). Primary percutaneous coronary intervention (PCI) was confirmed as the gold-standard therapy for STEMI, whereas thrombolysis can be helpful when the catheterization laboratory is not available or timely primary PCI cannot be achieved.[76]

For patients with COVID-19 and ischemic stroke, the use of thrombolysis and thrombectomy should be continued. There are some difficulties in managing neurologic rehabilitation, mostly related to organizational issues and risk of infection.[77]

Acute limb thrombosis associated with COVID-19 is characterized by greater clot burden and increased rate of amputation and death.[78] As for myocardial infarction and ischemic stroke, treatment involves prompt intervention, characterized first by therapeutic anticoagulation, preferably with UFH, and then by an assessment based on the stability and viability of the limb on the most appropriate approach.

COAGULOPATHY AND VACCINES

A turning point in the fight against COVID-19 has been the development of vaccines, whose efficacy, especially against severe forms of the disease, and safety profile has led to a rapid "conditional marketing authorization" by the main regulatory agencies.[79]

Abnormal activation of the coagulation system has been implicated in the pathogenesis of some severe adverse reactions related to the administration of anti–COVID-19 vaccines. After the marketing authorization, there have been increasing reports, albeit rare, of thrombotic complications at unusual sites, associated with thrombocytopenia, arising mainly after the administration of viral vector vaccines (Vaxzevria by AstraZeneca AB and COVID-19 Vaccine Janssen by Janssen-Cilag International NV). The incidence of this complication, named Vaccine-associated Immune Thrombosis and Thrombocytopenia (VITT) syndrome, remains largely unknown and appears to be between 1 in 125,000 and 1 in 1,000,000.[80]

In April 2021, the New England Journal of Medicine reports a total of 39 cases of thrombosis, observed after administration of the Vaxzevria vaccine, in different descriptive studies.[81–83] Clinical manifestations appear between 5 and 24 days after the first administration of the Astra-Zeneca serum. The affected population is predominantly female with an age of less than 50 years. In some cases (25.9%), affected women were using oral contraceptives. In most cases, thrombosis involved cerebral veins, although cases of involvement of the splanchnic venous district and PE have been described. Of note, severe thrombocytopenia (platelet count <25,000/mm^3) was present in 52.6% of the cases evaluated. The concomitance of thrombocytopenia and thrombosis suggested an autoimmune mechanism in the pathogenesis of the syndrome. A German group led by Andreas Greinacher shed light on the pathogenesis of VITT, highlighting its similarities to the condition known as HIT.[84] HIT is due to the formation of autoantibodies directed against a complex epitope formed by platelet-derived factor 4 (PF4) and heparin or another polyanionic molecule. These autoantibodies can bind the Fcγlla receptor (FcRγlla) present at the platelet surface causing intense intravascular platelet activation and aggregation.[85] They have also been found in VITT, even in the absence of previous heparin exposure.[81] The cause of the formation of these antibodies in patients with VITT is unclear.

Cases of platelet count reduction associated with bleeding in the absence of thrombotic phenomena have been described in persons vaccinated with mRNA vector vaccines (Comirnaty by BioNTech Manufacturing GmbH and COVID-19 Vaccine Moderna by Moderna Biotech Spain, SL). Although it is not yet clear whether there is a causal link between this condition and the vaccine, an autoimmune-type mechanism has been hypothesized here too.[86]

SUMMARY

Coagulopathy is common in acute sepsis. However, hypercoagulability associated with SARS-CoV-2 infection has peculiar features.

COVID-19 is associated with a high rate of thrombotic complications, mainly in the venous district. The "thromboinflammation" that characterizes the disease is evident in the alterations of laboratory parameters and some clinical manifestations characterized by a high mortality rate. Numerous clinical trials are ongoing to define the best preventive and therapeutic strategy in the management of thrombosis from COVID-19.

CLINICS CARE POINTS

- In the management of patients with COVID-19, attention must be paid to the occurrence of arterial and venous thromboembolic complications, which appear to be frequently associated with the disease
- COVID-19 is associated with changes in coagulation parameters, which are more evident in severe forms of the disease (increased D-dimer, lengthening of PT and INR, thrombocytopenia, and shortening or sometimes lengthening of aPTT).
- The diagnosis of thrombotic complications such as DVT or PE cannot be derived solely from laboratory parameters but needs to be correlated with symptoms and must be supported by imaging methods such as CT angiography or ultrasound. Some scoring systems can be useful (see **Table 1**)
- Current recommendations do not indicate antithrombotic prophylaxis in all COVID-19 patients. However, in subjects at high risk of VTE (immobility, procoagulative status, and previous VTE), antithrombotic prophylaxis should be considered.
- Low-molecular-weight heparin at prophylactic dosage should be considered in all patients (including noncritically ill) who require hospital admission for COVID-19 infection in the absence of any contraindications.
- The rare cases of thrombotic complications related to the administration of anti–COVID-19 vaccines, especially those using a viral vector, should not cast doubt on the advantages of vaccination. Epidemiologic data on adverse reactions and an understanding of the pathogenetic mechanisms may be helpful in limiting the incidence of such complications.

DISCLOSURE

The authors have nothing to disclose.

REFERENCES

1. Clerkin KJ, Fried JA, Raikhelkar J, et al. COVID-19 and cardiovascular disease. Circulation 2020; 141(20):1648–55.
2. Madjid M, Safavi-Naeini P, Solomon SD, et al. Potential effects of coronaviruses on the cardiovascular system: a review. 2020. JAMA Cardiol 2020;5(7): 831–40.

3. Driggin E, Madhavan MV, Bikdeli B, et al. Cardiovascular considerations for patients, health care workers, and health systems during the COVID-19 pandemic 2020;75:21.

4. Iba T, Levy JH, Levi M, et al. Coagulopathy in COVID-19. J Thromb Haemost 2020;18:2103–9.

5. Han H, Yang L, Liu R, et al. Prominent changes in blood coagulation of patients with SARS-CoV-2 infection. Clin Chem Lab Med CCLM 2020;58:1116–20.

6. Gerotziafas GT, Catalano M, Colgan M-P, et al, Scientific Reviewer Committee. Guidance for the management of patients with vascular disease or cardiovascular risk factors and COVID-19: position paper from VAS-European independent Foundation in Angiology/vascular medicine. Thromb Haemost 2020;120:1597–628.

7. Edler C, Schröder AS, Aepfelbacher M, et al. Dying with SARS-CoV-2 infection—an autopsy study of the first consecutive 80 cases in Hamburg, Germany. Int J Legal Med 2020;134:1275–84.

8. Ranucci M, Ballotta A, Di Dedda U, et al. The procoagulant pattern of patients with COVID-19 acute respiratory distress syndrome. J Thromb Haemost 2020;18:1747–51.

9. Guan W, Ni Z, Hu Y, et al. Clinical characteristics of coronavirus disease 2019 in China. N Engl J Med 2020;382:1708–20.

10. Dolhnikoff M, Duarte-Neto AN, Almeida Monteiro RA, et al. Pathological evidence of pulmonary thrombotic phenomena in severe COVID-19. J Thromb Haemost 2020;18:1517–9.

11. Carsana L, Sonzogni A, Nasr A, et al. Pulmonary post-mortem findings in a series of COVID-19 cases from northern Italy: a two-centre descriptive study. Lancet Infect Dis 2020;20:1135–40.

12. Menter T, Haslbauer JD, Nienhold R, et al. Postmortem examination of COVID-19 patients reveals diffuse alveolar damage with severe capillary congestion and variegated findings in lungs and other organs suggesting vascular dysfunction. Histopathology 2020;77:198–209.

13. Goshua G, Pine AB, Meizlish ML, et al. Endotheliopathy in COVID-19-associated coagulopathy: evidence from a single-centre, cross-sectional study. Lancet Haematol 2020;7:e575–82.

14. Jose RJ, Manuel A. COVID-19 cytokine storm: the interplay between inflammation and coagulation. Lancet Respir Med 2020;8:e46–7.

15. Panigada M, Bottino N, Tagliabue P, et al. Hypercoagulability of COVID-19 patients in intensive care unit: a report of thromboelastography findings and other parameters of hemostasis. J Thromb Haemost 2020;18:1738–42.

16. Escher R, Breakey N, Lämmle B. Severe COVID-19 infection associated with endothelial activation. Thromb Res 2020;190:62.

17. Gu SX, Tyagi T, Jain K, et al. Thrombocytopathy and endotheliopathy: crucial contributors to COVID-19 thromboinflammation. Nat Rev Cardiol 2021;18:194–209.

18. Cui S, Chen S, Li X, et al. Prevalence of venous thromboembolism in patients with severe novel coronavirus pneumonia. J Thromb Haemost 2020;18:1421–4.

19. Zhang L, Feng X, Zhang D, et al. Deep vein thrombosis in hospitalized patients with COVID-19 in Wuhan, China: prevalence, risk factors, and outcome. Circulation 2020;142:114–28.

20. Nahum J, Morichau-Beauchant T, Daviaud F, et al. Venous thrombosis among critically ill patients with coronavirus disease 2019 (COVID-19). JAMA Netw Open 2020;3:e2010478.

21. Koupenova M, Freedman JE. Platelets and immunity: going viral. Arterioscler Thromb Vasc Biol 2020;40:1605–7.

22. Manne BK, Denorme F, Middleton EA, et al. Platelet gene expression and function in patients with COVID-19. Blood 2020;136:1317–29.

23. Fitch-Tewfik JL, Flaumenhaft R. Platelet granule exocytosis: a comparison with chromaffin cells. Front Endocrinol, 2013;4(77).

24. Sut C, Tariket S, Aubron C, et al. The non-hemostatic aspects of transfused platelets. Front Med 2018;5:42.

25. Tyagi T, Ahmad S, Gupta N, et al. Altered expression of platelet proteins and calpain activity mediate hypoxia-induced prothrombotic phenotype. Blood 2014;123:1250–60.

26. Ackermann M, Verleden SE, Kuehnel M, et al. Pulmonary vascular endothelialitis, thrombosis, and angiogenesis in covid-19. N Engl J Med 2020;383:120–8.

27. Hoffmann M, Kleine-Weber H, Schroeder S, et al. SARS-CoV-2 cell entry depends on ACE2 and TMPRSS2 and is blocked by a clinically proven Protease inhibitor. Cell 2020;181:271–80.e8.

28. Perdomo J, Leung HHL, Ahmadi Z, et al. Neutrophil activation and NETosis are the major drivers of thrombosis in heparin-induced thrombocytopenia. Nat Commun 2019;10:1322.

29. Pine AB, Meizlish ML, Goshua G, et al. Circulating markers of angiogenesis and endotheliopathy in COVID-19. Pulm Circ 2020;10. 204589402096654.

30. Della Rocca DG, Magnocavallo M, Lavalle C, et al. Evidence of systemic endothelial injury and microthrombosis in hospitalized COVID-19 patients at different stages of the disease. J Thromb Thrombolysis 2021;51:571–6.

31. Lakatta EG, Levy D. Arterial and cardiac aging: major Shareholders in cardiovascular disease enterprises: Part II: the aging Heart in health: links to Heart disease. Circulation 2003;107:346–54.

32. Bikdeli B, Madhavan MV, Jimenez D, et al. COVID-19 and thrombotic or thromboembolic disease:

implications for prevention, antithrombotic therapy, and follow-up. J Am Coll Cardiol 2020;75:2950–73.

33. Obi AT, Barnes GD, Wakefield TW, et al. Practical diagnosis and treatment of suspected venous thromboembolism during COVID-19 pandemic. J Vasc Surg Venous Lymphat Disord 2020;8:526–34.

34. Lippi G, Favaloro EJ. D-Dimer is associated with severity of coronavirus disease 2019: a pooled analysis. Thromb Haemost 2020;120:876–8.

35. Lippi G, Plebani M, Henry BM. Thrombocytopenia is associated with severe coronavirus disease 2019 (COVID-19) infections: a meta-analysis. Clin Chim Acta 2020;506:145–8.

36. Gao Y, Li T, Han M, et al. Diagnostic utility of clinical laboratory data determinations for patients with the severe COVID-19. J Med Virol 2020;92:791–6.

37. Huang C, Wang Y, Li X, et al. Clinical features of patients infected with 2019 novel coronavirus in Wuhan, China. The Lancet 2020;395:497–506.

38. Lippi G, Salvagno GL, Ippolito L, et al. Shortened activated partial thromboplastin time: causes and management. Blood Coagul Fibrinolysis 2010;21: 459–63.

39. Tang N, Li D, Wang X, et al. Abnormal coagulation parameters are associated with poor prognosis in patients with novel coronavirus pneumonia. J Thromb Haemost 2020;18:844–7.

40. Levi M, Toh CH, Thachil J, et al. Guidelines for the diagnosis and management of disseminated intravascular coagulation. Br J Haematol 2009;145:24–33.

41. Ramacciotti E, Agati LB, Aguiar VCR, et al. Zika and Chikungunya virus and risk for venous thromboembolism. Clin Appl Thromb 2019;25. 107602961882118.

42. Smither S, O'Brien L, Eastaugh L, et al. Haemostatic changes in five patients infected with Ebola virus. Viruses 2019;11:647.

43. Zhang Y, Xiao M, Zhang S, et al. Coagulopathy and antiphospholipid antibodies in patients with Covid-19. N Engl J Med 2020;382:e38.

44. Mendoza-Pinto C, García-Carrasco M, Cervera R. Role of infectious diseases in the antiphospholipid syndrome (including its Catastrophic variant). Curr Rheumatol Rep 2018;20:62.

45. Abdel-Wahab N, Talathi S, Lopez-Olivo MA, et al. Risk of developing antiphospholipid antibodies following viral infection: a systematic review and meta-analysis. Lupus 2018;27:572–83.

46. Salluh JIF, Soares M, Meis ED. Antiphospholipid antibodies and multiple organ failure in critically ill cancer patients. Clinics 2009;64:79–82.

47. Jaff MR, McMurtry MS, Archer SL, et al. Management of massive and submassive pulmonary embolism, iliofemoral deep vein thrombosis, and chronic thromboembolic pulmonary hypertension: a scientific statement from the American Heart association. Circulation 2011;123:1788–830.

48. Klok FA, Kruip MJHA, van der Meer NJM, et al. Confirmation of the high cumulative incidence of thrombotic complications in critically ill ICU patients with COVID-19: an updated analysis. Thromb Res 2020;191:148–50.

49. Grillet F, Behr J, Calame P, et al. Acute pulmonary embolism associated with COVID-19 pneumonia detected with pulmonary CT angiography. Radiology 2020;296:E186–8.

50. Lodigiani C, Iapichino G, Carenzo L, et al. Venous and arterial thromboembolic complications in COVID-19 patients admitted to an academic hospital in Milan, Italy. Thromb Res 2020;191:9–14.

51. Fischer EA, Kinnear B, Sall D, et al. Hospitalist-operated compression ultrasonography: a point-of-care ultrasound study (HOCUS-POCUS). J Gen Intern Med 2019;34:2062–7.

52. Kwong JC, Schwartz KL, Campitelli MA, et al. Acute myocardial infarction after laboratory-confirmed influenza infection. N Engl J Med 2018;378:345–53.

53. Corrales-Medina VF, Madjid M, Musher DM. Role of acute infection in triggering acute coronary syndromes. Lancet Infect Dis 2010;10:83–92.

54. Bangalore S, Sharma A, Slotwiner A, et al. ST-segment elevation in patients with covid-19 — a case series. N Engl J Med 2020;382:2478–80.

55. Perini P, Nabulsi B, Massoni CB, et al. Acute limb ischaemia in two young, non-atherosclerotic patients with COVID-19. The Lancet 2020;395:1546.

56. Tan Y-K, Goh C, Leow AST, et al. COVID-19 and ischemic stroke: a systematic review and meta-summary of the literature. J Thromb Thrombolysis 2020;50:587–95.

57. Cantador E, Núñez A, Sobrino P, et al. Incidence and consequences of systemic arterial thrombotic events in COVID-19 patients. J Thromb Thrombolysis 2020;50:543–7.

58. Yang X, Yu Y, Xu J, et al. Clinical course and outcomes of critically ill patients with SARS-CoV-2 pneumonia in Wuhan, China: a single-centered, retrospective, observational study. Lancet Respir Med 2020;8:475–81.

59. Lippi G, Lavie CJ, Sanchis-Gomar F. Cardiac troponin I in patients with coronavirus disease 2019 (COVID-19): evidence from a meta-analysis. Prog Cardiovasc Dis 2020;63:390–1.

60. Yin S, Huang M, Li D, et al. Difference of coagulation features between severe pneumonia induced by SARS-CoV2 and non-SARS-CoV2. J Thromb Thrombolysis 2021;51:1107–10.

61. Talasaz AH, Sadeghipour P, Kakavand H, et al. Recent randomized trials of antithrombotic therapy for patients with COVID-19: JACC state-of-the-art review. J Am Coll Cardiol 2021;77:1903–21.

62. Fournier M, Faille D, Dossier A, et al. Arterial thrombotic events in Adult Inpatients with COVID-19. Mayo Clin Proc 2021;96:295–303.

63. Poterucha TJ, Libby P, Goldhaber SZ. More than an anticoagulant: do heparins have direct anti-inflammatory effects? Thromb Haemost 2017;117: 437–44.

64. Tang N, Bai H, Chen X, et al. Anticoagulant treatment is associated with decreased mortality in severe coronavirus disease 2019 patients with coagulopathy. J Thromb Haemost 2020;18:1094–9.

65. Thachil J, Tang N, Gando S, et al. ISTH interim guidance on recognition and management of coagulopathy in COVID-19. J Thromb Haemost 2020;18: 1023–6.

66. Hadid T, Kafri Z, Al-Katib A. Coagulation and anticoagulation in COVID-19. Blood Rev 2021;47:100761.

67. Paranjpe I, Fuster V, Lala A, et al. Association of treatment dose anticoagulation with in-hospital Survival among hospitalized patients with COVID-19. J Am Coll Cardiol 2020;76:122–4.

68. Lemos ACB, do Espírito Santo DA, Salvetti MC, et al. Therapeutic versus prophylactic anticoagulation for severe COVID-19: a randomized phase II clinical trial (HESACOVID). Thromb Res 2020;196:359–66.

69. Schindewolf M, Weitz JI. Broadening the categories of patients eligible for extended venous thromboembolism treatment. Thromb Haemost 2020;120: 014–26.

70. Available at: https://clinicaltrials.gov/ct2/show/NCT04662684. Accessed September 25, 2021.

71. Available at: https://clinicaltrials.gov/ct2/show/NCT04650087. Accessed September 25, 2021.

72. Etkin Y, Conway AM, Silpe J, et al. Acute arterial thromboembolism in patients with COVID-19 in the New York city area. Ann Vasc Surg 2021;70:290–4.

73. Choudry FA, Hamshere SM, Rathod KS, et al. High thrombus burden in patients with COVID-19 presenting with ST-segment elevation myocardial infarction. J Am Coll Cardiol 2020;76:1168–76.

74. De Luca G, Verdoia M, Cercek M, et al. Impact of COVID-19 pandemic on mechanical reperfusion for patients with STEMI. J Am Coll Cardiol 2020;76: 2321–30.

75. Zeng J, Huang J, Pan L. How to balance acute myocardial infarction and COVID-19: the protocols from Sichuan Provincial People's Hospital. Intensive Care Med 2020;46:1111–3.

76. Chieffo A, Stefanini GG, Price S, et al. EAPCI position statement on invasive management of acute coronary syndromes during the COVID-19 pandemic. Eur Heart J 2020;41:1839–51.

77. Venketasubramanian N, Anderson C, Ay H, et al. Stroke care during the COVID-19 pandemic: international expert panel review. Cerebrovasc Dis Basel Switz 2021;50:245–61.

78. Goldman IA, Ye K, Scheinfeld MH. Lower-extremity arterial thrombosis associated with COVID-19 is characterized by greater Thrombus burden and increased rate of amputation and death. Radiology 2020;297:E263–9.

79. Available at: https://www.ema.europa.eu/en/human-regulatory/overview/public-health-threats/coronavirus-disease-covid-19/treatments-vaccines-covid-19. Accessed September 28 2021.

80. Franchini M, Liumbruno GM, Pezzo M. COVID-19 vaccine-associated immune thrombosis and thrombocytopenia (VITT): Diagnostic and therapeutic recommendations for a new syndrome. Eur J Haematol 2021;107:173–80.

81. Greinacher A, Thiele T, Warkentin TE, et al. Thrombotic thrombocytopenia after ChAdOx1 nCov-19 vaccination. N Engl J Med 2021;384:2092–101.

82. Schultz NH, Sørvoll IH, Michelsen AE, et al. Thrombosis and thrombocytopenia after ChAdOx1 nCoV-19 vaccination. N Engl J Med 2021;384:2124–30.

83. Scully M, Singh D, Lown R, et al. Pathologic antibodies to platelet factor 4 after ChAdOx1 nCoV-19 vaccination. N Engl J Med 2021;384:2202–11.

84. Oldenburg J, Klamroth R, Langer F, et al. Diagnosis and management of vaccine-related thrombosis following AstraZeneca COVID-19 vaccination: guidance statement from the GTH. Hämostaseologie. 2021;41:184–9.

85. Linkins L-A. Heparin induced thrombocytopenia. BMJ 2015;350:g7566.

86. Lee E, Cines DB, Gernsheimer T, et al. Thrombocytopenia following Pfizer and Moderna SARS-CoV -2 vaccination. Am J Hematol 2021;96:534–7.

87. Ortega-Paz L, Capodanno D, Montalescot G, et al. Coronavirus Disease 2019–Associated Thrombosis and Coagulopathy: Review of the Pathophysiological Characteristics and Implications for Antithrombotic Management [cited 2021 Jul 15];10. J Am Heart Assoc 2021. Available at: https://www.ahajournals.org/doi/10.1161/JAHA.120.019650.

Prevalence and Clinical Implications of COVID-19 Myocarditis

Cristina Chimenti, MD, PhD[a,b,*], Michele Magnocavallo, MD[a],
Federico Ballatore, MD[a], Federico Bernardini, MD[a], Maria Alfarano, MD[a],
Domenico G. Della Rocca, MD, PhD[c], Paolo Severino, MD, PhD[a],
Carlo Lavalle, MD[a], Fedele Francesco, MD[a], Andrea Frustaci, MD[a,b]

KEYWORDS

• COVID-19 • Myocarditis • Myocardial damage • Arrhythmias • Vascular damage • SARS-CoV-2

KEY POINTS

- Cardiac involvement is frequent in patients with COVID-19, and myocarditis represents one of the most recurrent clinical manifestations.
- Pathophysiology of myocarditis is still understood; direct viral damage or cell-mediated cytotoxicity are the 2 likely mechanisms.
- Cardiac magnetic resonance (CMR) represents the most important diagnostic tool, and diffuse edema may be considered the only CMR hallmark of COVID-19 myocarditis.
- The management of COVID-19 myocarditis is firstly finalized to provide supportive care for heart failure and prevention of lethal cardiac arrhythmias.

INTRODUCTION

In December 2019 the first case of coronavirus disease 2019 (COVID-19) was described in Wuhan, China, in a patient complaining of flulike symptoms.[1] The pathogen has been recognized as a novel enveloped RNA β-coronavirus, named severe acute respiratory syndrome coronavirus 2 (SARS-CoV-2).

The clinical manifestations of COVID-19 are widely variable ranging from asymptomatic infection to multiorgan failure and death. Although the clinical course of SARS-CoV-2 infection is mostly characterized by respiratory involvement, ranging from mild influenzalike illness to acute respiratory distress syndrome, it soon became evident that COVID-19 affects multiple organ systems, including the cardiovascular system.[2–4] Overall, up to 30% of hospitalized patients have evidence of myocardial injury, which is associated with a greater need for mechanical ventilatory support and higher in-hospital mortality.[5,6] Cardiovascular manifestations include acute coronary syndrome, atrial and ventricular arrhythmias, myocarditis, and cardiogenic shock.[3] In particular, myocarditis is a well-recognized severe complication of COVID-19 and is associated with fulminant cardiogenic shock and sudden cardiac death.[7–9] The pathophysiology of cardiac injury remains poorly understood, and the management and outcomes of myocarditis are not yet clarified. Thus, the authors present a comprehensive review about COVID-19–related myocarditis, describing clinical characteristics, diagnostic workup, and management.

Funded by: CRUI2020.
[a] Department of Cardiovascular/Respiratory Diseases, Nephrology, Anesthesiology, and Geriatric Sciences, Policlinico Umberto I, Sapienza University of Rome, Rome, Italy; [b] Cellular and Molecular Cardiology Lab, IRCCS L. Spallanzani, Rome 00149, Italy; [c] Texas Cardiac Arrhythmia Institute, St. David's Medical Center, 3000 North IH-35, Suite 720, Austin, TX 78705, USA
* Corresponding author. Department of Cardiovascular/Respiratory Diseases, Nephrology, Anesthesiology, and Geriatric Sciences, Policlinico Umberto I, Sapienza University of Rome, Rome, Italy.
E-mail address: cristina.chimenti@uniroma1.it

Card Electrophysiol Clin 14 (2022) 53–62
https://doi.org/10.1016/j.ccep.2021.11.001
1877-9182/22/© 2021 Elsevier Inc. All rights reserved.

EPIDEMIOLOGY OF COVID-19–RELATED MYOCARDITIS

The annual incidence of acute myocarditis from all causes is approximately 22 cases per 100,000 population, with heart failure (HF) occurring in 0.5% to 4.0% of these cases.[10] The true prevalence of myocarditis among patients with COVID-19 is difficult to establish, because the early reports often lacked the specific diagnostic modalities to assess myocarditis, and the circulating biomarkers reflecting myocardial injury can also be related to nonprimary myocardial damage (multiorgan failure, hypoxia, hypoperfusion, and activation of hemostasis).[11]

Overall, several studies report that myocardial injury occurs in 15% to 27.8% of severe COVID-19 pneumonia cases.[12–14] In addition, COVID-19–related myocarditis are also described in patients without prior pneumonia, indicating the probability of late onset of cardiovascular complications, even in those with mild symptoms.[15,16] Otherwise, diffuse myocardial injury was also detected in the early stage of COVID-19–recovered patients who had no active cardiac symptoms.[17]

IMMUNOLOGIC AND PATHOPHYSIOLOGICAL MECHANISMS

SARS-CoV-2 is a β-coronavirus whose genome consists of single-stranded RNA with positive polarity that belongs to the Coronaviridae family. The virus invades the human host cell by binding with high affinity to the angiotensin-converting enzyme 2 (ACE-2) receptor. ACE-2 can be found on the ciliated columnar epithelial cells of the respiratory tract, type II pneumocytes, and cardiomyocytes. Therefore, this mechanism seems to be the pathway of SARS-CoV-2 infection of the human heart, especially in case of HF, as ACE-2 is upregulated.[18] After penetration, viral RNA enters the cell nucleus for replication inducing human immunologic response to the virus.[19]

The mechanism of heart damage remains poorly understood, and several mechanisms have been proposed to explain the underlying pathophysiology of COVID-19–related acute myocarditis.[20] Among them, the main theories are the following (Fig. 1):

a. *Myocardial damage due to the direct viral action*: SARS-CoV-2 invades cells by binding to ACE-2 receptors, which are expressed in human myocardium.[21] Despite that nowadays it is still unclear if SARS-CoV-2 is directly associated to cardiomyocyte infection and damage. Indeed, although myocarditis has been clearly recognized at endomyocardial biopsy (EMB) or autopsy, there is no current evidence of myocarditis directly produced by cardiomyocyte infection due to the SARS-CoV-2 in humans,[8,22–24] and the associated lymphocytic myocarditis may be related to the inflammatory reaction induced by cytokines[25] or by extrapulmonary migration of infected alveolar macrophages.

b. *Via cell-mediated cytotoxicity*: activated CD8 T lymphocytes migrate to the heart and cause myocardial inflammation, inducing the cytokine release syndrome, a severe inflammatory response resulting in hypoxia and apoptosis of cardiomyocytes. This cytokine storm is proposed as the main mechanism underlying COVID-19–induced acute fulminant myocarditis.[21,26] Substantial evidence suggest that elevated serum level of interleukin (IL)-6 is present in patients with COVID-19, especially in those with severe presentations.[27] As a matter of fact, IL-6 seems to be the central mediator of cytokine storm, in which it coordinates the proinflammatory responses from immune cells, including the T-lymphocytes.[28] This process causes T-lymphocyte activation and a further release of inflammatory cytokines, which stimulate more T-lymphocytes, leading to a positive feedback loop of immune activation and myocardial damage.[29] Furthermore, IL-6 might cause a displacement of plakoglobin, a desmosomal protein, that could be arrhythmogenic due to the deposition of fibrous tissue.[30]

c. *Interferon-mediated hyperactivation* of the innate and adaptive immune system has also been proposed, especially in pediatric myocarditis COVID-19 related.[31]

Most probably, as proposed by Esfandiarei and colleagues, the pathophysiology of viral myocarditis is a miscellaneous of direct viral cell injury and T-lymphocyte–mediated cytotoxicity, which can be augmented by the cytokine storm syndrome.[32] Furthermore, cardiotoxic antiviral therapies may play a role in the genesis of myocardial inflammation, and a drug-induced myocarditis should also be considered.[33,34]

CLINICAL PRESENTATION

Clinical presentation of SARS-CoV-2 myocarditis could be very different: some patients may present relatively mild symptoms, such as fatigue and dyspnea, whereas others may complain of chest pain or chest tightness.[15,20] Otherwise, many patients show symptoms of tachycardia and acute-onset

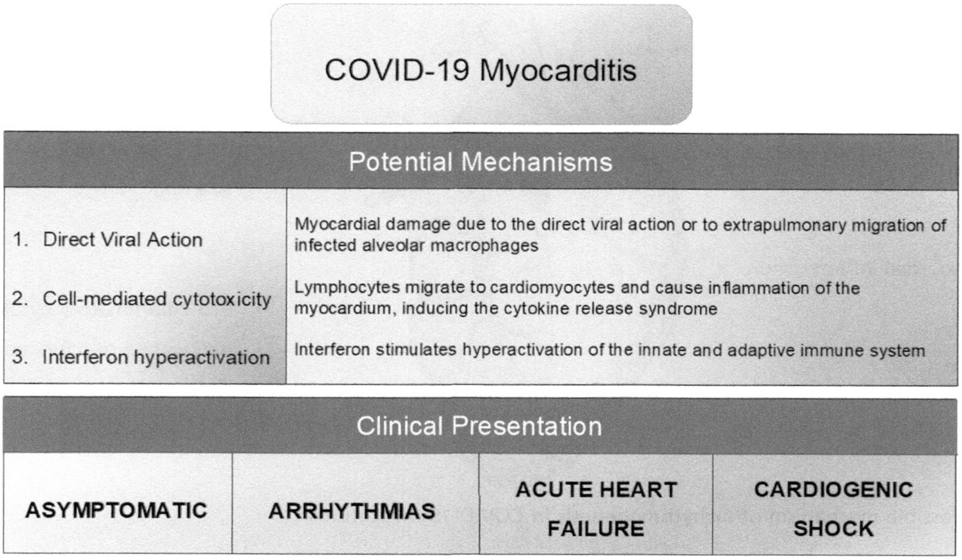

COVID-19 Myocarditis		
Potential Mechanisms		
1. Direct Viral Action	Myocardial damage due to the direct viral action or to extrapulmonary migration of infected alveolar macrophages	
2. Cell-mediated cytotoxicity	Lymphocytes migrate to cardiomyocytes and cause inflammation of the myocardium, inducing the cytokine release syndrome	
3. Interferon hyperactivation	Interferon stimulates hyperactivation of the innate and adaptive immune system	
Clinical Presentation		
ASYMPTOMATIC	ARRHYTHMIAS	ACUTE HEART FAILURE	CARDIOGENIC SHOCK

Fig. 1. Physiopathogenesis and clinical presentation of COVID-19 myocarditis.

HF until to cardiogenic shock or sudden cardiac death.[35–38] The early signs of fulminant myocarditis usually look similar to those of sepsis: hyperpiesia with low pulse pressure, cold or mottled extremities, and sinus tachycardia. Fulminant myocarditis is also frequently associated with ventricular arrhythmias because massive myocardial necrosis may generate some micro-reentry circuits and induce an electrolyte imbalance that triggers malignant tachycardia.[39–41] Overall, cardiac arrhythmias are frequently seen in patients with COVID-19 affected by myocarditis: several studies reported an incidence of cardiac arrhythmias between 15% and 20%.[42,43] The exact nature of the arrhythmias was not clearly reported but it has been speculated that their possible pathophysiology could include direct injury to cardiomyocytes and conduction system, ischemia from microvascular disease, reentrant arrhythmias due to myocardial fibrosis or scars, and proinflammatory cytokines predisposing to arrhythmogenicity (**Fig. 2**).[19,41,44]

DIAGNOSIS

In patients with COVID-19, the criteria for the diagnosis of myocarditis are the same as in other patients. However, the diagnostic pathway may be different because it is conditioned, first of all, by the need to protect all health care operators from the risk of SARS-CoV-2 infection.[45] In **Fig. 3** we provide a flow-chart for the diagnosis of COVID-19 myocarditis, considering troponin assessment as the first step in the diagnostic work up, because

it can be easily performed and its level is usually elevated in COVID-19–related myocarditis.[6,15] However, even in the presence of normal troponin if clinical suspicion of myocarditis is strong, cardiologic examinations should be performed. A fundamental step in the diagnostic process is the exclusion of obstructive coronary artery disease because high troponin level could be the result of exacerbation of patient's subclinical coronary artery disease due to inflammatory state, which increases cardiac oxygen demand. The oxygen supply–demand mismatch could in turn precipitate ischemia, resulting in type 2 myocardial infarction.[38,46,47]

Electrocardiographic (ECG) changes are not pathognomonic in myocarditis, because a variety of ECG patterns from sinus tachycardia and ectopic beats to ST elevation and T-wave inversion have been described.[48–50] Other ECG abnormalities, including new-onset bundle branch block, QT prolongation, pseudoinfarct pattern, and bradyarrhythmia with advanced atrioventricular nodal block, can be observed in myocarditis.

Transthoracic echocardiography is the first imaging technique performed and can be coupled with pulmonary ultrasound evaluation.[51] Global and regional ventricular systolic dysfunctions are not specific markers of acute myocarditis: ventricular dysfunction could be due to several other cardiac diseases, and, on the other hand, patients with myocarditis may have a normal left ventricular function. In addition, the possibility of a preexisting ventricular dysfunction should be always taken into consideration, especially if the patient has

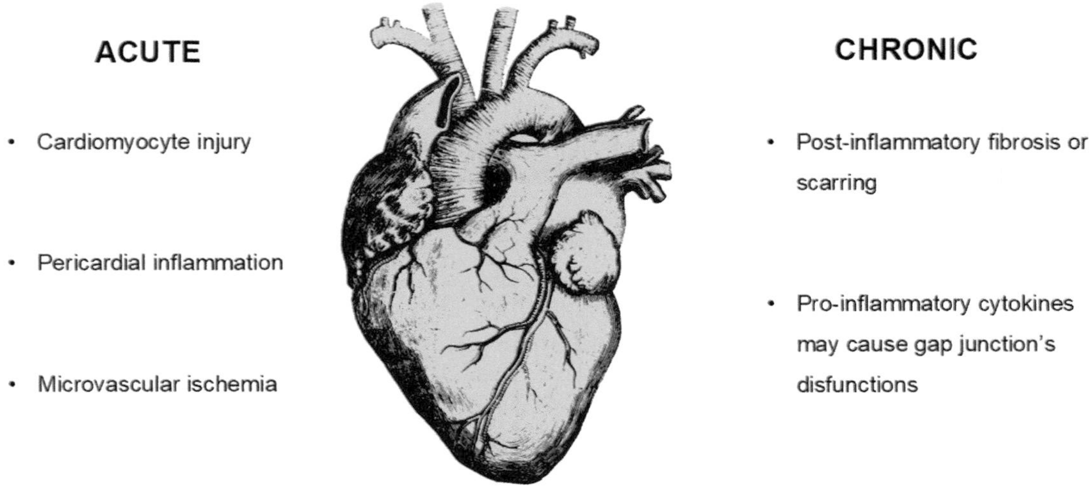

ACUTE

- Cardiomyocyte injury

- Pericardial inflammation

- Microvascular ischemia

CHRONIC

- Post-inflammatory fibrosis or scarring

- Pro-inflammatory cytokines may cause gap junction's disfunctions

Fig. 2. Possible mechanism of arrhythmogenesis in COVID-19 myocarditis.

known cardiovascular risk factors. Echocardiography also has prognostic implications; patients with marked reduction in right ventricular function have an increased risk of death.[52]

Thus, in patients with elevated troponin the presence of normal ECG and echocardiogram cannot exclude completely a COVID-19 myocarditis, and a close cardiologic follow-up should be performed.

Cardiac magnetic resonance (CMR) should be always performed in case of abnormal ECG and/or echocardiogram, and the findings should be interpreted according to the revised Lake Louise consensus criteria.[53,54] In clinically stable patients, both CMR and coronary computed tomography could be theoretically performed for myocarditis diagnosis in a radiology section dedicated to patients with COVID-19. CMR is used in patients

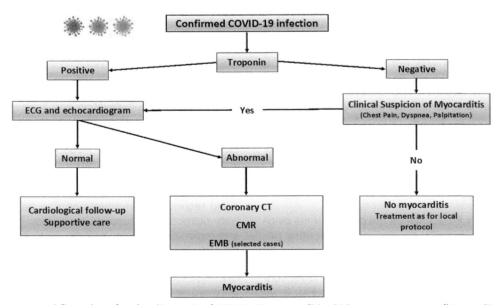

Fig. 3. Proposed flow-chart for the diagnosis of COVID-19 myocarditis. CAD, coronary artery disease; CMR, cardiac magnetic resonance; COVID-19, coronavirus disease 2019; CTA, computed tomography angiography; EMB, endomyocardial biopsy; PCI, percutaneous coronary intervention.

with COVID-19 to assess biventricular function, the pattern of edema and inflammation within the myocardium, and the presence of pericardial involvement. The common imaging findings on CMR included increased T1 and T2 mapping values and edema on T2/STIR sequences.[55] Diffuse edema may be considered the only CMR hallmark of COVID-19 myocarditis because late gadolinium enhancement (LGE) may be completely absent or minimal, revealing unremarkable myocyte necrosis.[56] LGE was seen in less than half of the patients, and if present, LGE was detected in the subepicardial location.[55] The presence of biventricular dysfunction; the detection of patchy, midwall, septal, or inferior LGE enhancement; and its persistence over 3 months have been associated with adverse cardiac events including sudden cardiac death and heart transplantation.[57–59]

In selected cases with CMR that suggest myocarditis, an EMB may be performed. The consensus paper from the American Heart Association/American College of Cardiology recommended EMB preferably in new-onset HF with hemodynamic instability or in life-threatening arrhythmias to establish the specific therapy.[60,61] Although EMB is definitive for the diagnosis, it is rarely used in patients with COVID-19 probably to limit spread of the infection to medical workers. When performed, the EMB showed scattered myocyte necrosis and CD4 and CD8 lymphocytes near vascular structures in patients with mild troponin elevation,[55,62] whereas patients with more severe clinical presentations had interstitial inflammation and vasculitis of intramural vessels represented by T-lymphocytes and CD68+ macrophages, associated to foci of necrosis (**Fig. 4**). The macrophage infiltration was seen to correlate with the elevated systemic levels of proinflammatory cytokines. Although coronary involvement was uncommon, endotheliitis was commonly encountered because virus showed tropism for endothelial cells.[36,63]

TREATMENT

The management of COVID-19 myocarditis is firstly finalized to provide a comprehensive management of HF.[64] However, a prompt treatment of respiratory symptoms aiming to promote viral clearance may have an additional benefit of reducing subsequent cardiovascular complications.

Management of Heart Failure

Patients who develop HF from COVID-19 myocarditis should be treated with guideline-directed medical therapy, including ACE inhibitors, angiotensin receptor blockers (ARBs), or angiotensin receptor-neprilysin inhibitors (ARNi), β-blockers and diuretics.[65] Because of their mechanism of action, there was initial concern that treating patients with COVID-19 with ACEi, ARB, and ARNi would worsen clinical outcomes. Thus, several recent observational studies showed that there was no significant difference between patients treated with ACEi or ARB and those who discontinue these medications and, therefore, is generally recommended to initiate or continue these drugs during and beyond the disease.[66,67]

In patients with fulminant myocarditis and cardiogenic shock, the administration of inotropes and/or vasopressors is recommended in the acute phase and mechanical circulatory support in the longer term.[68]

Appropriate management of cardiac arrhythmias related to COVID-19 myocarditis is crucial in mitigating patient's adverse health outcomes. Bradyarrhythmia may require temporary cardiac pacing, whereas tachyarrhythmias may respond to antiarrhythmic drugs. β-blockers may be considered for hemodynamically stable patients, whereas amiodarone is typically administered in the critically ill, although it can prompt QTc prolongation, especially when combined with azithromycin or hydroxychloroquine.[69–71] Alternatively, lidocaine infusion or oral flecainide may be considered.[72–74]

SARS-CoV-2 Viral Therapies

Therapies for SARS-CoV-2 have focused primarily on restoration of respiratory function, and there are little data to define therapeutic options in COVID-19 myocarditis. Different antiviral therapies were expected to be effective in hospitalized patients with COVID-19: remdesivir, hydroxychloroquine, and interferon beta-1a. Unfortunately, all these drugs had little or no effect on overall mortality, initiation of ventilation, and duration of hospital stay.[75,76] Moreover, many pharmacologic agents used empirically to treat COVID-19, especially hydroxychloroquine, may expose patients to an increased risk of cardiac arrhythmias: indeed, hydroxychloroquine may cause QTc interval prolongation, and its combination therapy with macrolides should be accompanied by QTc interval monitoring.[77]

Nonsteroidal antiinflammatory drugs are generally not indicated in myocarditis patients because they are the known cause of renal impairment and sodium retention, which could exacerbate acute ventricular dysfunction.[68]

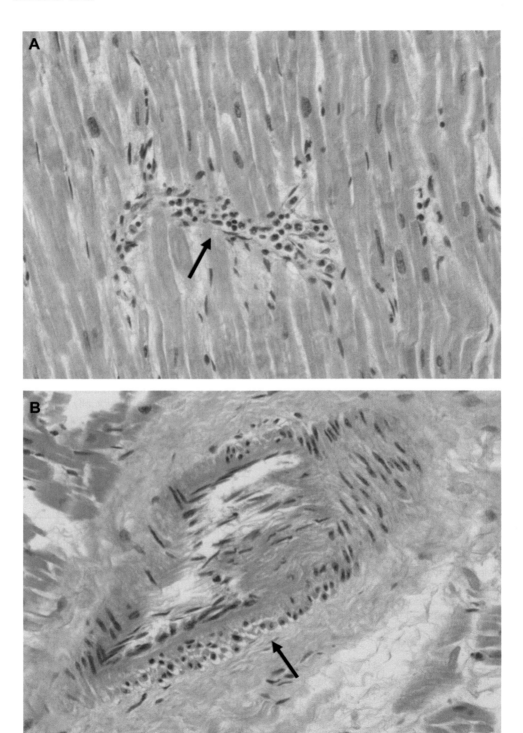

Fig. 4. Left ventricular endomyocardial biopsy of a patient with COVID-19 myocarditis. (*A*) Focal active myocarditis depicted by lymphomononuclear infiltrated (*arrows*) with necrosis of the adjacent cardiomyocytes (hematoxylin and eosin 10X magnification). (*B*) Myocarditis was associated with vasculitis of intramural vessels (hematoxylin and eosin 20X magnification).

Because cytokine release syndrome is a probable mechanism of injury in COVID-19 myocarditis, some investigators suggested to use antiinflammatory and anticytokine drugs such as high-dose steroids and intravenous immunoglobulins (IVIG).[78] However, the use of high-dose steroids in patients with COVID-19 has given conflicting results: if in a retrospective study there was an improvement of survival, another trial showed a reduction in viral clearance, increased risk of over infection, and mortality for all causes.[79–81] Overall, in patients hospitalized with COVID-19 the use of corticosteroid resulted in a clinical benefit only in those who were receiving invasive mechanical ventilation and oxygen therapy.[82]

Regarding purified IVIG, they gave encouraging result in a small group of 5 critical patients with COVID-19 without clinically suspected myocarditis but no additional evidence exists in patients with COVID-19–established myocarditis.[83] The immunomodulatory effects of IVIG are multifactorial, showing not only antiviral effects but also antiinflammatory effects by suppressing inflammatory cytokines.[84] Currently, the evidence does not support the routine use of IVIGs alone.

Several immune therapies have also been investigated, and agents targeting IL-6, such as tocilizumab, have also been evaluated in the REMAP-CAP study, showing promising results in critically ill patients.[85]

In summary, in patients with isolated SARS-CoV-2 myocarditis who are hospitalized, or hypoxemic, high-dose steroids may be reasonable, whereas it should be avoided in patients with less severe illness. Regarding targeted immunomodulatory therapy with IL-6 antagonists, additional data are needed to establish whether it can be recommended for SARS- CoV-2 myocarditis.

PROGNOSIS

Although there are very limited data about the clinical outcomes of COVID-19 myocarditis, it seems that most patients have a favorable prognosis.[56,86] The complexity of COVID-19 and the possibility to die of other reasons than cardiac involvement (acute severe respiratory distress, systemic embolism, multiorgan failure) should also be underlined. Overall, Shi and colleagues reported that patients with myocardial injury presented higher mortality rate than those without myocardial injury (51.2% vs 4.5%; $P < .001$), being an independent risk factor for mortality.[12] In addition, myocardial injury was associated with a higher incidence of severe respiratory distress (58.5% vs 14.7%), need of noninvasive (46.3% vs 3.9%) or invasive ventilation (22.0% vs 4.2%), and complications such as acute kidney injury (8.5% vs 0.3%) and coagulopathy (7.3% vs 1.8%).[12] Also, patients with an increase of troponin present higher levels of leukocytes, D-dimer, ferritin, and IL-6, portraying an important correlation between myocardial injury and inflammatory hyperactivity triggered by the viral infection. Raised troponin levels in COVID-19 are associated with worse outcome, but the specific prognostic role of myocarditis is unknown.[87]

In general, myocardial involvement in COVID-19 is associated with an increased mortality, but isolated myocarditis is not necessarily a marker of poor prognosis. However, given the paucity of published data and the inhomogeneity of the cases, conclusive assertion on prognosis cannot be made.

SUMMARY

Myocarditis is a common complication of COVID-19 infection. Direct viral damage or cell-mediated cytotoxicity are the 2 likely pathophysiological mechanisms. Although CMR represents the most important diagnostic tool because diffuse edema may be considered the only CMR hallmark of COVID-19 myocarditis, the definitive diagnosis of myocarditis is obtained via EMB. Treatment of myocarditis should be based on therapy for ventricular dysfunction and clinical status, including arrhythmias and HF, whereas high-dose steroids should be reserved to more compromised patients. Myocardial involvement in COVID-19 is associated with an increased mortality, but isolated myocarditis is not necessarily a marker of poor prognosis.

CLINICS CARE POINTS

- Myocarditis are very frequent among COVID-19 patients.
- A comprehensive diagnostic approach should be pursued in these patients.
- Endomyocardial biopsy is necessary to exclude other form of myocarditis.

DISCLOSURE

All authors have reported that they have no relationships relevant to the contents of this article to disclose.

REFERENCES

1. Zhu N, Zhang D, Wang W, et al. A novel coronavirus from patients with pneumonia in China, 2019. N Engl J Med 2020;382:727–33.
2. Chen N, Zhou M, Dong X, et al. Epidemiological and clinical characteristics of 99 cases of 2019 novel coronavirus pneumonia in Wuhan, China: a Descriptive study. Lancet 2020;395:507–13.
3. Madjid M, Safavi-Naeini P, Solomon SD, et al. Potential effects of coronaviruses on the cardiovascular system: a review. JAMA Cardiol 2020;5:831.
4. Della Rocca DG, Magnocavallo M, Lavalle C, et al. Evidence of systemic endothelial injury and microthrombosis in hospitalized COVID-19 patients at different stages of the disease. J Thromb Thrombolysis 2020. https://doi.org/10.1007/s11239-020-02330-1.
5. Lala A, Johnson KW, Januzzi JL, et al. Prevalence and impact of myocardial injury in patients hospitalized with COVID-19 infection. J Am Coll Cardiol 2020;76:533–46.
6. Richardson S, Hirsch JS, Narasimhan M, Crawford JM, McGinn T, Davidson KW, the Northwell COVID-19 Research Consortium, Barnaby DP, Becker LB, Chelico JD, et al. Presenting characteristics, comorbidities, and outcomes among 5700 patients hospitalized with COVID-19 in the New York city Area. JAMA 2020;323:2052.
7. Kesici S, Aykan HH, Orhan D, et al. Fulminant COVID-19-related myocarditis in an infant. Eur Heart J 2020;41:3021.
8. del Nonno F, Frustaci A, Verardo R, et al. Virus-negative myopericarditis in human coronavirus infection: report from an autopsy Series. Circ Heart Fail 2020;13. https://doi.org/10.1161/CIRCHEARTFAILURE.120.007636.
9. Daniels CJ, Rajpal S, Greenshields JT, et al. Prevalence of clinical and subclinical myocarditis in Competitive Athletes with recent SARS-CoV-2 infection: results from the big ten COVID-19 cardiac registry. JAMA Cardiol 2021. https://doi.org/10.1001/jamacardio.2021.2065.
10. Vos T, Barber RM, Bell B, et al. Global, regional, and National incidence, prevalence, and years lived with disability for 301 acute and chronic diseases and injuries in 188 countries, 1990–2013: a systematic analysis for the global burden of disease study 2013. Lancet 2015;386:743–800.
11. Siripanthong B, Nazarian S, Muser D, et al. Recognizing COVID-19–related myocarditis: the possible pathophysiology and proposed guideline for diagnosis and management. Heart Rhythm 2020;17:1463–71.
12. Shi S, Qin M, Shen B, et al. Association of cardiac injury with mortality in hospitalized patients with COVID-19 in Wuhan, China. JAMA Cardiol 2020;5:802. https://doi.org/10.1001/jamacardio.2020.0950.
13. Guo T, Fan Y, Chen M, et al. Cardiovascular implications of fatal outcomes of patients with coronavirus disease 2019 (COVID-19). JAMA Cardiol 2020;5:811. https://doi.org/10.1001/jamacardio.2020.1017.
14. Maestrini V, Birtolo LI, Francone M, et al. Cardiac involvement in consecutive unselected hospitalized COVID-19 population: in-hospital evaluation and one-Year follow-up. Int J Cardiol 2021;339:235–42.
15. Inciardi RM, Lupi L, Zaccone G, et al. Cardiac involvement in a patient with coronavirus disease 2019 (COVID-19). JAMA Cardiol 2020;5:819. https://doi.org/10.1001/jamacardio.2020.1096.
16. Kim I-C, Kim JY, Kim HA, et al. COVID-19-Related myocarditis in a 21-year-old female patient. Eur Heart J 2020;41:1859.
17. Puntmann VO, Carerj ML, Wieters I, et al. Outcomes of cardiovascular magnetic resonance imaging in patients recently recovered from coronavirus disease 2019 (COVID-19). JAMA Cardiol 2020;5:1265.
18. Kawakami R, Sakamoto A, Kawai K, et al. Pathological evidence for SARS-CoV-2 as a cause of myocarditis. J Am Coll Cardiol 2021;77:314–25.
19. Bhatla A, Mayer MM, Adusumalli S, et al. COVID-19 and cardiac arrhythmias. Heart Rhythm 2020;17:1439–44.
20. Carretta DM, Silva AM, D'Agostino D, et al. Cardiac involvement in COVID-19 patients: a contemporary review. Infect Dis Rep 2021;13:494–517.
21. Ranard LS, Fried JA, Abdalla M, et al. Approach to acute cardiovascular complications in COVID-19 infection. Circ Heart Fail 2020;13. https://doi.org/10.1161/CIRCHEARTFAILURE.120.007220.
22. Escher F, Pietsch H, Aleshcheva G, et al. Detection of viral SARS-CoV-2 genomes and histopathological changes in endomyocardial Biopsies. ESC Heart Fail 2020;7:2440–7.
23. Lindner D, Fitzek A, Bräuninger H, et al. Association of cardiac infection with SARS-CoV-2 in confirmed COVID-19 autopsy cases. JAMA Cardiol 2020;5:1281.
24. Basso C, Leone O, Rizzo S, et al. Pathological features of COVID-19-associated myocardial injury: a multicentre cardiovascular pathology study. Eur Heart J 2020;41:3827–35.
25. Sala S, Peretto G, Gramegna M, et al. Acute myocarditis presenting as a reverse tako-tsubo syndrome in a patient with SARS-CoV-2 respiratory infection. Eur Heart J 2020;41:1861–2.
26. Gralinski LE, Baric RS. Molecular pathology of emerging coronavirus infections. J Pathol 2015;235:185–95.
27. Coomes EA, Haghbayan H. Interleukin-6 in Covid-19: a Systematic review and meta-analysis. Rev Med Virol 2020;30:1–9.
28. Lee DW, Gardner R, Porter DL, et al. Current concepts in the diagnosis and management of cytokine release syndrome. Blood 2014;124:188–95.
29. Fox SE, Akmatbekov A, Harbert JL, et al. Pulmonary and cardiac Pathology in African American patients with COVID-19: an autopsy Series from new Orleans. Lancet Respir Med 2020;8:681–6.

0. Asimaki A, Tandri H, Duffy ER, et al. Altered desmosomal proteins in granulomatous myocarditis and potential pathogenic links to arrhythmogenic right ventricular cardiomyopathy. Circ Arrhythm Electrophysiol 2011;4:743–52.

1. McMurray JC, May JW, Cunningham MW, et al. Multisystem inflammatory syndrome in Children (MIS-C), a Post-viral myocarditis and systemic vasculitis—a critical review of its pathogenesis and treatment. Front Pediatr 2020;8:626182.

2. Esfandiarei M, McManus BM. Molecular biology and pathogenesis of viral myocarditis. Annu Rev Pathol Mech Dis 2008;3:127–55.

3. Alijotas-Reig J, Esteve-Valverde E, Belizna C, et al. Immunomodulatory therapy for the management of severe COVID-19. Beyond the anti-viral therapy: a comprehensive review. Autoimmun Rev 2020;19: 102569. https://doi.org/10.1016/j.autrev.2020.102569.

4. Russell K, Eriksen M, Aaberge L, et al. A novel clinical method for quantification of regional left ventricular pressure–strain loop area: a non-invasive Index of myocardial work. Eur Heart J 2012;33: 724–33.

5. Zeng J-H, Liu Y-X, Yuan J, et al. First case of COVID-19 complicated with fulminant myocarditis: a case report and insights. Infection 2020;48:773–7.

6. Frustaci A, Francone M, Verardo R, et al. Virus-negative necrotizing coronary vasculitis with aneurysm formation in human SARS-CoV-2 infection. Infect Dis Rep 2021;13:597–601.

7. Lavalle C, Ricci RP, Santini M. Atrial tachyarrhythmias and cardiac resynchronisation therapy: clinical and therapeutic implications. Heart 2010;96:1174–8.

8. Di Biase L, Romero J, Du X, et al. Catheter ablation of ventricular tachycardia in ischemic cardiomyopathy: impact of concomitant amiodarone therapy on short- and long-term clinical outcomes. Heart Rhythm 2021;18:885–93.

9. Di Biase L, Romero J, Zado ES, et al. Variant of ventricular outflow tract ventricular arrhythmias requiring ablation from multiple sites: intramural origin. Heart Rhythm 2019;16:724–32.

0. Lakkireddy DR, Chung MK, Gopinathannair R, et al. Guidance for cardiac Electrophysiology during the COVID-19 Pandemic from the heart Rhythm Society COVID-19 Task Force; Electrophysiology section of the American College of Cardiology; and the Electrocardiography and arrhythmias Committee of the Council on clinical Cardiology, American heart association. Heart Rhythm 2020;17:e233–41.

1. Wu C-I, Postema PG, Arbelo E, et al. SARS-CoV-2, COVID-19, and Inherited arrhythmia syndromes. Heart Rhythm 2020;17:1456–62.

2. Coromilas EJ, Kochav S, Goldenthal I, et al. Worldwide Survey of COVID-19–associated arrhythmias. Circ Arrhythmia Electrophysiol 2021;14. https://doi.org/10.1161/CIRCEP.120.009458.

43. Liu K, Fang Y-Y, Deng Y, et al. Clinical characteristics of novel coronavirus cases in Tertiary hospitals in Hubei Province. Chin Med J 2020;133:1025–31.

44. Della Rocca DG, Pepine CJ. Endothelium as a Predictor of adverse outcomes: Endothelium as a Predictor of adverse outcomes. Clin Cardiol 2010;33:730–2.

45. Mele D, Flamigni F, Rapezzi C, et al. Myocarditis in COVID-19 patients: current Problems. Intern Emerg Med 2021;16:1123–9.

46. Clerkin KJ, Fried JA, Raikhelkar J, et al. COVID-19 and cardiovascular disease. Circulation 2020;141: 1648–55.

47. Chimenti C, Scopelliti F, Vulpis E, et al. Increased Oxidative stress Contributes to cardiomyocyte dysfunction and death in patients with Fabry disease Cardiomyopathy. Hum Pathol 2015;46: 1760–8.

48. Forleo GB, Della Rocca DG, Papavasileiou LP, et al. Predictive value of Fragmented QRS in primary prevention Implantable Cardioverter Defibrillator Recipients with left ventricular dysfunction. J Cardiovasc Med 2011;12:779–84.

49. Romero J, Alviz I, Parides M, et al. T-wave inversion as a manifestation of COVID-19 infection: a case Series. J Interv Card Electrophysiol 2020;59:485–93.

50. Chen Q, Xu J, Gianni C, et al. Simple Electrocardiographic criteria for Rapid Identification of Wide QRS Complex tachycardia: the new Limb Lead Algorithm. Heart Rhythm 2020;17:431–8.

51. D'Andrea Antonello, Di Giannuario Giovanna, Marrazzo Gemma, et al. L'imaging integrato nel percorso del paziente con COVID-19: dalla diagnosi, al monitoraggio clinico, alla prognosi. Giornale Italiano di Cardiologia 2020. https://doi.org/10.1714/3343. 33132.

52. Szekely Y, Lichter Y, Taieb P, et al. Spectrum of cardiac manifestations in COVID-19: a Systematic echocardiographic study. Circulation 2020;142:342–53.

53. Friedrich MG, Sechtem U, Schulz-Menger J, et al. Cardiovascular magnetic resonance in myocarditis: a JACC white paper. J Am Coll Cardiol 2009;53: 1475–87. https://doi.org/10.1016/j.jacc.2009.02.007.

54. Ferreira VM, Schulz-Menger J, Holmvang G, et al. Cardiovascular magnetic resonance in Nonischemic myocardial inflammation. J Am Coll Cardiol 2018;72: 3158–76.

55. Ojha V, Verma M, Pandey NN, et al. Cardiac magnetic resonance imaging in coronavirus disease 2019 (COVID-19): a Systematic review of cardiac magnetic resonance imaging findings in 199 patients. J Thorac Imaging 2021;36:73–83.

56. Esposito A, Palmisano A, Natale L, et al. Cardiac magnetic resonance Characterization of myocarditis-like acute cardiac syndrome in COVID-19. JACC: Cardiovasc Imaging 2020;13:2462–5.

57. Caforio ALP, Calabrese F, Angelini A, et al. A Prospective study of biopsy-Proven myocarditis:

prognostic relevance of clinical and Aetiopathogenetic Features at diagnosis. Eur Heart J 2007;28:1326–33.

58. Grün S, Schumm J, Greulich S, et al. Long-term follow-up of biopsy-Proven viral myocarditis. J Am Coll Cardiol 2012;59:1604–15.

59. Gräni C, Eichhorn C, Bière L, et al. Prognostic value of cardiac magnetic resonance tissue Characterization in risk Stratifying patients with suspected myocarditis. J Am Coll Cardiol 2017;70:1964–76.

60. Cooper LT, Baughman KL, Feldman AM, et al. The role of endomyocardial biopsy in the management of cardiovascular disease: a scientific statement from the American heart association, the American College of Cardiology, and the European society of Cardiology. Circulation 2007;116:2216–33.

61. Tarantino N, Della Rocca DG, De Leon De La Cruz NS, et al. Catheter ablation of life-threatening ventricular arrhythmias in Athletes. Medicina 2021;57:205.

62. Fox SE, Li G, Akmatbekov A, et al. Unexpected features of cardiac pathology in COVID-19 infection. Circulation 2020;142:1123–5.

63. Fox SE, Lameira FS, Rinker EB, et al. Cardiac endotheliitis and multisystem inflammatory syndrome after COVID-19. Ann Intern Med 2020;173:1025–7.

64. Agdamag ACC, Edmiston JB, Charpentier V, et al. Update on COVID-19 myocarditis. Medicina (Kaunas) 2020;56:E678.

65. McDonagh TA, Metra M, Adamo M, et al. 2021 ESC guidelines for the diagnosis and treatment of acute and chronic heart failure. Eur Heart J 2021;42:3599–726.

66. Lopes RD, Macedo AVS, de Barros E Silva PGM, et al. Effect of discontinuing vs continuing angiotensin-converting enzyme inhibitors and angiotensin II receptor blockers on days alive and out of the hospital in patients admitted with COVID-19: a randomized clinical trial. JAMA 2021;325:254.

67. Mehra MR, Desai SS, Kuy S, et al. Retraction: cardiovascular disease, drug therapy, and mortality in covid-19. N Engl J Med 2020;382:2582.

68. Kociol RD, Cooper LT, Fang JC, et al. Recognition and initial management of fulminant myocarditis: a scientific statement from the American heart association. Circulation 2020;141. https://doi.org/10.1161/CIR.0000000000000745.

69. Mercuro NJ, Yen CF, Shim DJ, et al. Risk of QT interval prolongation associated with use of hydroxychloroquine with or without concomitant azithromycin among hospitalized patients Testing positive for coronavirus disease 2019 (COVID-19). JAMA Cardiol 2020;5:1036.

70. Gasperetti A, Biffi M, Duru F, et al. Arrhythmic safety of hydroxychloroquine in COVID-19 patients from different clinical Settings. EP Europace 2020;22:1855–63.

71. Frustaci A, Morgante E, Antuzzi D, et al. Inhibition cardiomyocyte lysosomal activity in hydroxychlor quine cardiomyopathy. Int J Cardiol 2012;15 117–9.

72. Lavalle C, Magnocavallo M, Straito M, et al. Fleca nide how and when: a practical guide in supraven tricular arrhythmias. JCM 2021;10:1456.

73. Lavalle C, Trivigno S, Vetta G, et al. Flecainide ventricular arrhythmias: from old myths to new pe spectives. JCM 2021;10:3696.

74. Della Rocca DG, Tarantino N, Trivedi C, et al. Non-pu monary vein triggers in nonparoxysmal atrial fibrillatio implications of pathophysiology for Catheter Ablatio J Cardiovasc Electrophysiol 2020;31:2154–67.

75. WHO Solidarity trial Consortium Repurposed An viral drugs for Covid-19 — Interim WHO Solidari trial results. N Engl J Med 2021;384:497–511.

76. The RECOVERY Collaborative group effect of h droxychloroquine in hospitalized patients wi Covid-19. N Engl J Med 2020;383:2030–40.

77. Piro A, Magnocavallo M, Della Rocca DG, et a Management of cardiac Implantable Electronic D vice follow-up in COVID-19 Pandemic: Lesson Learned during Italian Lockdown. J Cardiovas Electrophysiol 2020;14755. jce.

78. Mehta P, McAuley DF, Brown M, et al. COVID-1 Consider cytokine storm syndromes and Immun suppression. Lancet 2020;395:1033–4.

79. Wu C, Chen X, Cai Y, et al. Risk factors associated wi acute respiratory distress syndrome and death in p tients with coronavirus disease 2019 pneumonia Wuhan, China. JAMA Intern Med 2020;180:934.

80. Russell CD, Millar JE, Baillie JK. Clinical evidenc does not support corticosteroid treatment for 201 NCoV Lung injury. Lancet 2020;395:473–5.

81. Frustaci A, Chimenti C. Immunosuppressive therap in myocarditis. Circ J 2014;79:4–7.

82. The RECOVERY Collaborative group Dexametha sone in hospitalized patients with Covid-19. N En J Med 2021;384:693–704.

83. Shen C, Wang Z, Zhao F, et al. Treatment of 5 cri cally ill patients with COVID-19 with Convalesce Plasma. JAMA 2020;323:1582.

84. Kow CS, Hasan SS. Glucocorticoid versus immun globulin in the treatment of COVID-19-associate fulminant myocarditis. Infection 2020;48:805–6.

85. The REMAP-CAP Investigators interleukin-6 rece tor antagonists in critically ill patients with Covi 19. N Engl J Med 2021;384:1491–502.

86. Sawalha K, Abozenah M, Kadado AJ, et al. Syste atic review of COVID-19 related myocarditis: I sights on management and outcome. Cardiovas Revascularization Med 2021;23:107–13.

87. Castiello T, Georgiopoulos G, Finocchiaro G, et COVID-19 and myocarditis: a systematic revie and overview of current challenges. Heart Fail R 2021. https://doi.org/10.1007/s10741-021-10087-9

Electrocardiographic Features of Patients with COVID-19: An Updated Review

Jorge Romero, MD, FHRS[a], Mohamed Gabr, MD[a], Juan Carlos Diaz, MD[b],
Sutopa Purkayastha, MD[a], Maria T. Gamero, MD[a], Olga Reynbakh, MD[a],
Jose Matias, MD[a], Isabella Alviz, MD[a], Alejandro Velasco, MD[a],
Domenico G. Della Rocca, MD[c], Sanghamitra Mohanty, MD[c],
Aung Lin, MD[a], Fengwei Zou, MD[a], Andrea Natale, MD[c],
Luigi Di Biase, MD, PhD[a],*

KEYWORDS

• COVID 19 • ECG • Electrocardiography

KEY POINTS

- Electrocardiographic (ECG) changes seen in association with COVID-19 include QRS axis changes, conduction abnormalities, and ST segment and T-wave changes.
- QTc interval changes, commonly described at the beginning of the pandemic, are now less frequently seen due to increased awareness for the need of QTc monitoring and avoidance of QT prolonging drugs, resulting in a reduction of possibly fatal arrhythmic events.
- Atrial and ventricular arrhythmias are more common in critically ill patients with COVID-19, with atrial fibrillation being the most commonly reported rhythm disturbance.
- The mechanisms for the development of ECG changes and arrhythmias are multifactorial.

INTRODUCTION

Since its declaration as a pandemic more than year ago, the novel severe acute respiratory syndrome coronavirus-2 (SARS-CoV-2) has affected more than 180 million people worldwide and sadly claimed more than 4 million lives, including more than 33 million cases and 600,000 deaths in the United States alone. SARS-CoV-2's effects continue to unravel, as it affects nations worldwide, health care systems and economies adjust to battle it, and the daily livelihoods of billions of people and patients are touched. In addition, patients, a lot of whom suffer from the aftermaths and morbidity inflicted by the disease, are chronically influenced by SARS-CoV-2, and this has led to escalation of efforts by physicians and researchers worldwide for the development of treatments and vaccinations to limit its extension and decrease morbidity and mortality.[1] Subsequently, the abundance of data regarding disease processes, disease associations, different manifestations, and pathophysiology of the COVID-19 has improved our understanding of the disease and how to approach it. Varying mortality rates have been described, ranging from 1 per 100,000 to 100 per 100,000,[2] and several factors have been associated with higher morbidity and mortality,

Funding: none.
[a] Cardiac Arrhythmia Center, Division of Cardiology, Department of Medicine, Montefiore-Einstein Center for Heart and Vascular Care, Albert Einstein College of Medicine, Bronx, NY, USA; [b] Clinica Las Americas, Medellin, Colombia; [c] Texas Cardiac Arrhythmia Institute, St. David's Medical Center, Austin, TX, USA
* Corresponding author. Cardiac Arrhythmia Center, Division of Cardiology, Department of Medicine, Montefiore–Einstein Center for Heart and Vascular Care, Albert Einstein College of Medicine, 111 East 210th Street, Bronx, NY 10467.
E-mail address: dibbia@gmail.com

Card Electrophysiol Clin 14 (2022) 63–70
https://doi.org/10.1016/j.ccep.2021.10.006

including previously known comorbidities, advanced age, obesity, or male gender.[3,4]

Different organ systems are involved as a result of SARS-CoV-2 infection including pulmonary involvement with hypoxemic respiratory (which is commonly responsible for deterioration and mortality), renal involvement,[5,6] multisystem inflammatory syndromes,[7] and a wide array of cardiac manifestations. Numerous studies have described the existence of cardiac involvement in patients infected with SARS-CoV-2, with increased mortality.[8–10] In addition, cardiac involvement has been demonstrated on cardiac imaging such as magnetic resonance imaging (MRI) in patients who recovered from COVID-19,[11] and by evidence of right ventricular (RV) dysfunction, left ventricular (LV) systolic dysfunction, and LV diastolic dysfunction on transthoracic echocardiography.[12] In addition, cardiac manifestations have been described in electrocardiographic (ECG) features that include cardiac arrhythmias, ST segment changes, and QT prolongation.

METHODS

In this review, the authors aim to summarize ECG characteristics in patients with COVID-19, the pathophysiology behind them, and their implications. They performed a database search of PubMed, Embase, and Cochrane Central Register of Clinical Trials for articles using the keywords "COVID" OR "coronavirus" OR "SARS-CoV-2" OR "SARS" AND "electrocardiogram" OR "EKG" OR "ECG" OR "arrhythmia." The search yielded 1433 results. Prospective and retrospective studies, systematic reviews, meta-analyses, case reports and series, narrative reviews, letters, and clinical guidelines were reviewed. The authors reviewed relevant articles for data to comprehensively discuss and describe the ECG features encountered thus far in COVID-19.

DISCUSSION
Axis, QRS, and Atrioventricular Conduction

Changes to cardiac axis, in addition to QRS complex morphology and atrioventricular (AV) conduction, have been reported with SARS-CoV-2 (Fig. 1). In order to assess ECG changes in patients admitted with COVID-19, McCullough and colleagues analyzed ECGs of 756 patients in a New York City hospital.[13] On review, 19.3% had an abnormal QRS axis: 13.8% in the form of left axis deviation and 5.5% in the form of right or right superior axis deviation. In other studies, ECG changes in the form of right axis deviation have been reported in patients with evidence of RV

strain, such as in patients with extensive pulmo nary disease and pneumonia, or when pulmonar embolism occurs as a complication of COVID-1 with significant clot burden.[14] Conduction abno malities were also noted in 11.8% of the cohor with left bundle branch block in 1.5% of the pa tients, right bundle branch block in 7.8%, an nonspecific intraventricular block in 2.5%. In add tion, 29% of patients had nonspecific repolariza tion abnormalities. AV block was observed 2.6%, with the majority (2.5%) being first-degre AV block. Atrial premature contractions occurre in 7.7% and ventricular premature contractions 3.4%. Atrial premature contractions (OR 2.3 95% CI 1.27-4.21, P = .006), repolarization abno malities (OR 2.31, 95% CI 1.27-4.21, P = .006 and right bundle branch block/intraventricula block (OR 2.61, 95% CI 1.32-5.18, P = .00 were predictors of increased mortality.[13]

ST Segment and T-Wave Changes

ST segment deviations, whether elevations or de pressions, are amongst the ECG changes presen in patients infected with SARS-CoV-2. (Fig. 2A case series of patients admitted with COVID-1 reviewed 18 patients who either presented wit ST segment elevations or developed ST elevation during hospitalizations. After stratification base on echocardiographic features and wall motio peak troponin levels, and patient symptom 50% of these patients underwent coronary ang ography, of which 67% were found to hav obstructive coronary disease. Forty-four perce of the patients described in the cohort were diag nosed with myocardial infarction, whereas 56 were thought to have noncoronary-relate myocardial injury.[15] In addition to myocard infarction, ST segment changes have been attrib uted to myocardial injury in the form of myocardi or microthrombi.[16–18] For instance, in patients wit COVID-19 myocarditis, nearly 50% of patients ha ST-segment elevation on ECG. Echocardiograph features observed in these patients include card omegaly or increased wall thickness, decrease ejection fraction, or global hypokinesis in near two-thirds of patients,[19] as well as late gadoliniu enhancement on MRI in all patients. In additio surrogates of myocardial injury such as troponin and T are frequently elevated.

Furthermore, in a recent case series, the autho described the finding of new T-wave inversio (TWI) in patients with SARS-CoV-2 and its assoc ation with increased mortality, need for intubatio and mechanical ventilation, particularly in patient with concomitant elevation of cardiac troponir (Fig. 2B, C).[20] In this study of 3225 patient

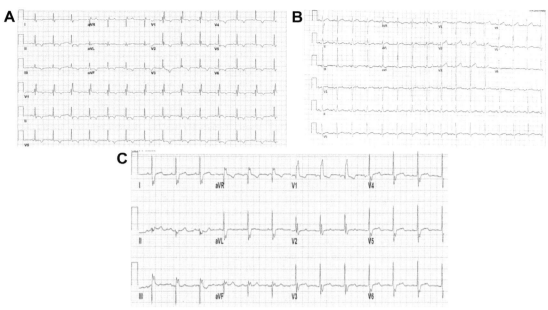

Fig. 1. Axis and QRS in patients with COVID-19. (*A*) Incomplete right bundle branch block. Diffuse T wave inversion involving septal, anterior, inferior and lateral leads is also observed; (*B*) right axis deviation; (*C*) left axis deviation. Right bundle branch block is also present.

admitted with COVID-19, 6% of patients had either new TWI or pseudonormalization, with 23% of these patients having concomitant troponin elevation. TWI were observed in the lateral leads (71%), anterior leads (64%), inferior leads (57%), and septal leads (26%). In addition, roughly one-quarter of the patients who had a transthoracic echocardiogram were found to have regional wall motion abnormalities, and mortality was 35%, 52%, and 80% if TWI were diffuse, accompanied by elevated troponin levels, or both, respectively. In addition, other studies have corroborated ST and T-wave changes and their relation to cardiac injury and mortality in COVID-19.[13,21] An analysis by Barman and colleagues of ECG findings in 219 patients admitted with COVID-19 based on

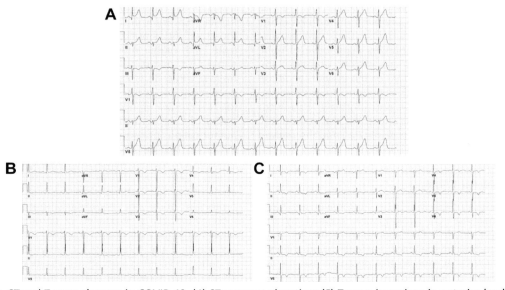

Fig. 2. ST and T-wave changes in COVID-19. (*A*) ST segment elevation; (*B*) T-wave inversions in anterior leads; (*C*) T-wave inversions in anterolateral leads.

clinical severity (95 severe and 124 nonsevere infection) revealed more frequent ST depressions (28% vs 14%), ST-T changes (36% vs 21%), and TWI (29% vs 16%) in patients with severe infection compared with nonsevere infection.[22]

Although the exact mechanisms of myocardial injury contributing to ST-segment and T-wave morphology changes are unknown, it is hypothesized that this occurs as a result of myocardial microthrombi formation (involving primarily capillaries, arterioles and small muscular arteries),[23] direct damage to the cardiomyocytes, systemic inflammatory response syndromes, cytokine-mediated responses by helper T cells, and interferon-mediated immune response. In addition, hypoxia as a result of COVID-19–associated respiratory failure and coronary plaque destabilization may be other contributors.[16] These theories are supported by evidence of myocyte necrosis and interstitial edema with predominant lymphocytic infiltration in an animal model of coronavirus infection, as well as endomyocardial biopsy in a human subject revealing interstitial and endocardial inflammation, and viral particle presence in interstitial cells with loss of cytoplasmic membrane integrity.[24,25] COVID-19 severity and the presence of cardiac injury defined as elevated high-sensitivity troponin I were found to be independent predictors of ECG changes in the form of ST segments and T-wave changes (odds ratio [OR] 1.87 and 3.32, respectively) in an analysis of patients with COVID-19.[22] In another study, the investigators conferred that the number of abnormal T waves was an indicator of myocardial injury (OR 2.36, 95% confidence interval [CI], 1.38–4.04, $P = .002$) and that the presence of T-wave changes in itself was a predictor of mortality (hazard ratio, 3.57 [1.40, 9.11], $P = .008$).[21] Moreover, ST segment/T-wave changes suggestive of right heart strain such as ST depressions or T-wave inversions in leads V1 to V3 or the inferior leads, or presence of the S1Q3T3 pattern, may correlate with disease outcomes and mortality. However, in a study of 15 patients with pulmonary embolism and COVID-19, only 1 patient (7%) had the pathognomonic pattern of S1Q3T3.[26]

QT Interval Changes

Previous studies with other coronaviruses have demonstrated QT prolongation caused by the infection itself.[25] QT interval prolongation has been particularly described extensively in patients with COVID-19, due to the potential risk for arrhythmias or torsades de pointes (TdP).[27] For instance, in an international multicenter registry that enrolled 110 patients, 14% of patients

developed QTc prolongation after 7 days of hospitalization (mean QTc increase 66 ± 2 msec, +16%, $P < .001$), with a 3.6% incidenc of life-threatening arrhythmias.[28] Independent predictors of QTc prolongation included older age higher basal heart rate, and treatment with dua antiviral therapy. In earlier stages of the pandemic concerns regarding QTc-prolonging drugs tha were believed to be beneficial for treatment c COVID-19, such as azithromycin, chloroquine hydroxychloroquine (HCQ), and lopinavir/ritonavir triggered calls for monitoring and caution while using these drugs.[29] In one study that included 9 patients with SARS-CoV-2 infection,[30] fc example, patients receiving concomitant azithromycin and HCQ were noted to have a greater me dian (interquartile range) change in QT interva compared with hydroxychloroquine alone (2 [10–40] vs 5.5 [−15.5 to 34.25] msec; respectively $P = .03$). In addition, seven patients (19%) wh received hydroxychloroquine alone develope prolonged QTc of greater than 500 msec and 3 pa tients (3%) had a QTc increase of 60 msec c more. Of those who received concomitant azithro mycin, 11 of 53 (21%) had prolonged QTc c 500 msec or more and 7 of 53 (13%) had a chang in QTc of 60 msec or more. Moreover, HCQ wa discontinued in one patient due to TdP.[30] Anothe study of 98 patients assessed critical QTc prolor gation, defined as maximum QTc greater than c equal to 500 ms (if QRS <120 ms) or QTc greate than or equal to 550 ms (if QRS ≥ 120 ms), an QTc increase of greater than or equal to 60 ms i patients receiving HCQ, azithromycin, or a comb nation of both. In this cohort, 12% of patients me the criteria for critical QTc prolongation, with higher incidence in patients taking combinatic therapy.[31] Additional studies described similar re sults, with higher mortality rates in patients wit either QTc greater than 500 ms or an increase c 60 ms[32] (Fig. 3). Consequently, this led to healt care systems using policies for baseline an follow-up ECG monitoring, remote and telemon toring of QTc, and the FDA granting emergenc authorization for the use of the KardiaMobile 6 (AliveCor, Inc) device for this purpose. Howeve more recent studies suggest that the QTc prolor gation seen with SARS-CoV-2 infection an some of the medications used in earlier treatmer protocols does not necessarily translate int higher mortality or incidence of cardiac arrhyth mias;[32] this may be due to the QTc prolongatio not meeting the threshold for arrhythmogenesi or better monitoring leading to cessation of drug when certain thresholds are met (QTc ≥ 500 m or increase in QTc interval ≥ 60 ms).[33] In additior with emerging evidence of lack of benefit of HC(

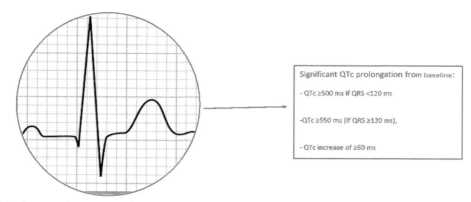

Fig. 3. QTc changes that warrant frequent QTc monitoring in SARS-CoV-2 infection.

and azithromycin, administration of these medications, particularly in combination, has been greatly limited.

Arrhythmias in COVID-19

Although sinus rhythm and sinus tachycardia remain the most common rhythms encountered in patients with COVID-19, cardiac arrhythmias, as other cardiac manifestations of COVID-19, have been of interest, given their relevance and possible effects on morbidity and mortality inflicted by the disease (**Fig. 4**A). Earlier data emerging from China[33] at the onset of the pandemic reported incidences of up to 17% of patients admitted with SARS-COV-2 infection having arrhythmias, higher rates of up to 44% in patients requiring intensive care unit (ICU) care, and around 7% of admitted patients having ventricular tachycardia or ventricular fibrillation. Subsequent data from 700 patients admitted in a US hospital, 11%

of which required ICU admission, reported 25 incident atrial fibrillation (AF) events, 10 nonsustained ventricular tachycardias (NSVTs), 9 clinically significant bradyarrhythmias, and 9 cardiac arrests—all the arrests occurred in ICU-admitted patients.[34] Furthermore, ICU admission was associated with arrhythmias such as incident AF and NSVT (OR 4.68 [95% confidence interval [CI] 1.66–13.18] and 8.92 [95% CI 1.73–46.06]; respectively), and in-hospital mortality only increased with cardiac arrests. Similarly, a meta-analysis of studies that included 5815 patients with COVID-19 reported an arrhythmia incidence of 9.3%,[35] and a Heart Rhythm Society survey of electrophysiologists worldwide reported that atrial fibrillation was the most commonly encountered arrhythmia (21%) by professionals treating patients with COVID-19.[36]

Multiple factors likely contribute to arrhythmias in patients affected by COVID-19. Acute myocardial injury occurring in some patients, can in itself trigger

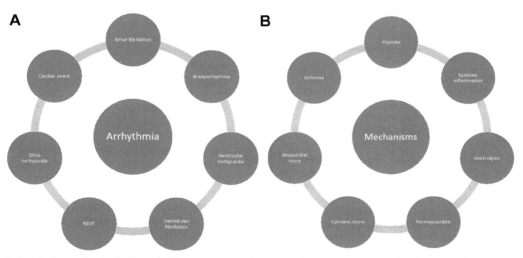

Fig. 4. (A) Arrhythmias in COVID-19; (B) mechanism of arrhythmias. NSVT, nonsustained ventricular tachycardia.

cardiac arrhythmias. In a study of 1284 patients with severe COVID-19, 170 patients had evidence of myocardial injury as evidenced by elevated cardiac troponin I, of which 26% had arrhythmias.[37] Conversely, in a meta-analysis that assessed the role of cardiac injury as a predictor of mortality and severe disease, incidence of new arrhythmias was found to be associated with higher risk of severe disease and the need for ICU admission (risk ratio 13, 95% CI 7.00–24.47, $P < .001$).[38] Moreover, hypoxia and electrolyte abnormalities may contribute to bradyarrhythmias, atrial fibrillation, and ventricular arrhythmias; and systemic inflammation, viral perimyocarditis, and proarrhythmogenicity induced by certain medications may predispose to atrial and ventricular arrhythmias (**Fig. 4**B). In addition, bradyarrhythmias, interestingly, have been suggested to be a possible sign associated with developing cytokine storm.[39]

SUMMARY

ECG features in patients with COVID-19 range from changes in morphologies of QRS complexes, ST segments, and T waves, to changes in cardiac axis, QTc interval, and cardiac arrhythmias, which may be atrial or ventricular in origin. Often, these findings are due to severe systemic illness inflicted by hypoxic injury, electrolyte abnormalities, endothelial or myocardial injury, microthrombi and plaque rupture, and cytokine storm. Knowledge of these ECG features, paired with patients' clinical status, cardiac imaging findings, and cardiac biomarkers, can assist clinicians in accurately assessing and tailoring care through an understanding of the underlying disease processes.

CLINICS CARE POINTS

- Clinicians should be cognizant of some of the reported ECG changes, such as abnormal QRS axis in nearly 20% of patients, conduction abnormalities in approximately 20%, AV block in about 2.6%, and premature beats in nearly 10% of patients.
- ST segment and T-wave changes in patients with COVID-19 can be due to myocardial infarction or myocardial injury secondary to myocarditis, inflammatory responses, or microthrombi and should therefore be interpreted in the correct clinical context, as they can be associated with illness severity and mortality.

- Baseline and follow-up ECG for QTc monitoring is suggested in hospitalized patients. Clinically significant QTc prolongation can be defined as intraventricular QTc of greater than or equal to 500 ms with a normal QRS interval, greater than or equal to 550 ms if QRS greater than or equal to 120 ms, or QTc increase of greater than or equal to 60 ms from baseline.
- Although sinus rhythm is the most common, nearly 9.3% of patients admitted with COVID-19 are reported to have arrhythmias, with atrial fibrillation being the most incident. Arrhythmias can be a sign of myocardial injury and increased disease severity, and the treatment focus should be on the underlying infection and any potential triggers.

ACKNOWLEDGMENTS

None

DISCLOSURE

Dr L. Di Biase is a consultant for Stereotaxis, Biosense Webster, Boston Scientific, and Abbott Medical and has received speaker honoraria/travel support from Medtronic, Atricure, Bristol Meyers Squibb, Pfizer, and Biotronik. Dr A. Natale is a consultant for Biosense Webster, Stereotaxis, and Abbott and has received speaker honoraria, travel support from Medtronic, Atricure, Biotronik, and Janssen. Remaining authors report no conflict of interest.

REFERENCES

1. Ferrari R, Maggioni AP, Tavazzi L, et al. The battle against COVID-19: mortality in Italy. Eur Heart J 2020;41(22):2050–2.
2. Bilinski A, Emanuel EJ. COVID-19 and excess all-cause mortality in the US and 18 comparison countries. JAMA 2020;324(20):2100–2.
3. Grasselli G, Zangrillo A, Zanella A, et al. Baseline characteristics and outcomes of 1591 patients infected with SARS-CoV-2 admitted to ICUs of the lombardy region, Italy. JAMA 2020;323(16): 1574–81.
4. Guzik TJ, Mohiddin SA, Dimarco A, et al. COVID-19 and the cardiovascular system: implications for risk assessment, diagnosis, and treatment options. Cardiovasc Res 2020;116(10):1666–87.
5. Bitencourt L, Pedrosa AL, Soares de Brito SBC, et al. COVID-19 and renal diseases: an update. Curr Drug Targets 2021;22(1):52–67.
6. Santoriello D, Khairallah P, Bomback AS, et al. Postmortem Kidney Pathology Findings in Patients with

COVID-19. J Am Soc Nephrol. 2020 Sep;31(9): 2158–67.

7. Morris SB, Schwartz NG, Patel P, et al. Case series of multisystem inflammatory syndrome in adults associated with SARS-CoV-2 infection - United Kingdom and United States, March-August 2020. MMWR Morb Mortal Wkly Rep 2020;69(40):1450–6.

8. Bonow RO, O'Gara PT, Yancy CW. Cardiology and COVID-19. JAMA 2020;324(12):1131–2.

9. Shi S, Qin M, Shen B, et al. Association of cardiac injury with mortality in hospitalized patients with COVID-19 in Wuhan, China. JAMA Cardiol 2020;5(7):802–10.

10. Santoso A, Pranata R, Wibowo A, et al. Cardiac injury is associated with mortality and critically ill pneumonia in COVID-19: a meta-analysis. Am J Emerg Med 2020;44:352–7.

11. Puntmann VO, Carerj ML, Wieters I, et al. Outcomes of cardiovascular magnetic resonance imaging in patients recently recovered from Coronavirus Disease 2019 (COVID-19). JAMA Cardiol 2020;5(11): 1265–73.

12. Szekely Y, Lichter Y, Taieb P, et al. Spectrum of cardiac manifestations in COVID-19: a systematic echocardiographic study. Circulation 2020;142(4): 342–53.

13. McCullough SA, Goyal P, Krishnan U, et al. Electrocardiographic findings in Coronavirus Disease-19: insights on mortality and underlying myocardial processes. J Card Fail 2020;26(7):626–32.

14. Elias P, Poterucha TJ, Jain SS, et al. The prognostic value of electrocardiogram at presentation to Emergency Department in patients with COVID-19. Mayo Clin Proc 2020;95(10):2099–109.

15. Bangalore S, Sharma A, Slotwiner A, et al. ST-segment elevation in patients with Covid-19 - a case series. N Engl J Med 2020;382(25):2478–80.

16. Babapoor-Farrokhran S, Gill D, Walker J, et al. Myocardial injury and COVID-19: possible mechanisms. Life Sci 2020;253:117723.

17. Castiello T, Georgiopoulos G, Finocchiaro G, et al. COVID-19 and myocarditis: a systematic review and overview of current challenges. Heart Fail Rev. 2021 Mar 24;1–11. https://doi.org/10.1007/s10741-021-10087-9. Epub ahead of print.

18. Guagliumi G, Sonzogni A, Pescetelli I, et al. Microthrombi and ST-segment-elevation myocardial infarction in COVID-19. Circulation 2020;142(8):804–9.

19. Kariyanna PT, Sutarjono B, Grewal E, et al. A systematic review of COVID-19 and myocarditis. Am J Med Case Rep 2020;8(9):299–305.

20. Romero J, Alviz I, Parides M, et al. T-wave inversion as a manifestation of COVID-19 infection: a case series. J Interv Card Electrophysiol 2020;59(3): 485–93.

21. Chen L, Feng Y, Tang J, et al. Surface electrocardiographic characteristics in coronavirus disease 2019: repolarization abnormalities associated with cardiac involvement. ESC Heart Fail 2020;7(6): 4408–15.

22. Barman HA, Atici A, Alici G, et al. The effect of the severity COVID-19 infection on electrocardiography. Am J Emerg Med 2020;46:317–22.

23. Pellegrini D, Kawakami R, Guagliumi G, et al. Microthrombi as a Major Cause of Cardiac Injury in COVID-19: A Pathologic Study. Circulation 2021 Mar 9;143(10):1031–42.

24. Tavazzi J, Pellegrini C, Maurelli M, et al. Myocardial localization of coronavirus in COVID-19 cardiogenic shock. Eur J Heart Fail. 2020 May;22(5):911–5.

25. Alexander LK, Keene BW, Yount BL, et al. ECG changes after rabbit coronavirus infection. J Electrocardiol 1999;32(1):21–32.

26. Kho J, Ioannou A, Van den Abbeele K, et al. Pulmonary embolism in COVID-19: clinical characteristics and cardiac implications. Am J Emerg Med 2020; 38(10):2142–6.

27. Jankelson L, Karam G, Becker ML, et al. QT prolongation, torsades de pointes, and sudden death with short courses of chloroquine or hydroxychloroquine as used in COVID-19: a systematic review. Heart Rhythm 2020;17(9):1472–9.

28. Santoro F, Monitillo F, Raimondo P, et al. QTc interval prolongation and life-threatening arrhythmias during hospitalization in patients with COVID-19. Results from a multi-center prospective registry [published online ahead of print, 2020 Oct 24]. Clin Infect Dis. 2020;ciaa1578. https://doi.org/10.1093/cid/ciaa1578.

29. Giudicessi JR, Noseworthy PA, Friedman PA, et al. Urgent guidance for navigating and circumventing the QTc-prolonging and torsadogenic potential of possible pharmacotherapies for Coronavirus Disease 19 (COVID-19). Mayo Clin Proc 2020;95(6): 1213–21.

30. Mercuro NJ, Yen CF, Shim DJ, et al. Risk of QT interval prolongation associated with use of hydroxychloroquine with or without concomitant azithromycin among hospitalized patients testing positive for Coronavirus Disease 2019 (COVID-19). JAMA Cardiol 2020;5(9):1036–41.

31. Ramireddy A, Chugh H, Reinier K, et al. Experience with hydroxychloroquine and azithromycin in the coronavirus disease 2019 pandemic: implications for QT interval monitoring. J Am Heart Assoc 2020; 9(12):e017144.

32. Hsia BC, Greige N, Quiroz JA, et al. QT prolongation in a diverse, urban population of COVID-19 patients treated with hydroxychloroquine, chloroquine, or azithromycin. J Interv Card Electrophysiol 2020;59(2): 337–45.

33. Chang D, Saleh M, Gabriels J, et al. Inpatient use of ambulatory telemetry monitors for COVID-19 patients treated with hydroxychloroquine and/or azithromycin. J Am Coll Cardiol 2020;75(23):2992–3.

34. Bhatla A, Mayer MM, Adusumalli S, et al. COVID-19 and cardiac arrhythmias. Heart Rhythm 2020;17(9): 1439–44.

35. Kunutsor SK, Laukkanen JA. Cardiovascular complications in COVID-19: a systematic review and meta-analysis. J Infect 2020;81(2):e139–41.

36. Gopinathannair R, Merchant FM, Lakkireddy DR, et al. COVID-19 and cardiac arrhythmias: a global perspective on arrhythmia characteristics and management strategies. J Interv Card Electrophysiol 2020;59(2):329–36.

37. Si D, Du B, Ni L, et al. Death, discharge and arrhythmias among patients with COVID-19 and cardiac injury. CMAJ 2020;192(28):E791–8.

38. Li X, Pan X, Li Y, et al. Cardiac injury associated with severe disease or ICU admission and death in hospitalized patients with COVID-19: a meta-analysis and systematic review. Crit Care. 2020 Jul 28;24(1):468.

39. Manolis AS, Manolis AA, Manolis TA, et al. COVID-19 infection and cardiac arrhythmias. Trends Cardiovasc Med 2020;30(8):451–60.

Echocardiography in COVID-19 Pandemic
Clinical Findings and the Importance of Emerging Technology

Alberto Barosi, MD[a],*, Luca Bergamaschi, MD[a], Ignazio Cusmano, MD[a], Alessio Gasperetti, MD[a,b], Marco Schiavone, MD[a], Elisa Gherbesi, MD[a]

KEYWORDS

• COVID-19 • Echocardiography • Myocardial strain • Ultramobile devices

ECHOCARDIOGRAPHY IN COVID-19 PATIENTS

Coronavirus disease 2019 (COVID-19) mainly affects the respiratory system,[1] but important amount of evidence has described cardiac involvement,[2,3] in up to 20% of patients,[4] besides collaterally leading toward a change in hospital admission patterns for other cardiac diseases.[5–7] Echocardiography, as a widely available, cost-effective tool for the evaluation of cardiac structure and function, can provide important information that can affect the management of COVID-19 patients, but considering the risk of equipment contamination and personnel exposure,[8] focused evaluations instead of complete echocardiograms and the use of portable devices easy to disinfect, are recommended.

The present review discusses the principal echocardiographic findings in COVID-19 patients (**Fig. 1**; **Table 1**), practical aspects, and the role of emerging technology.

LEFT AND RIGHT VENTRICLE: MAJOR FINDINGS

COVID-19 can cause a wide range of cardiac conditions, which include acute myocardial infarction,[9–11] takotsubo cardiomyopathy,[12] myocarditis,[13] arrhythmogenic,[14] thrombotic manifestations,[15] and potential drug-related effects,[16–18] as documented by several studies and early case reports.

However, the incidence of the cardiac involvement and the subsequent implications for treatment and resource allocation for the screening of these conditions are not well defined, but data confirmed that cardiac injury is associated with increased mortality in COVID-19.[19,20]

Regarding myocardial infarction, Stefanini and colleagues collected, in a national registry, 28 COVID-19 patients with ST-elevation myocardial infarction (STEMI): in approximately 40% of them, a culprit lesion was not detected by coronary angiography, pointing out the role of cytokine storm, hypoxic injury, coronary spasm, microthrombi, direct endothelial, or vascular injury. On echocardiography, about 80% of patients had localized left ventricular (LV) wall motion abnormalities, whereas left ventricular ejection fraction (LVEF) was less than 50% in about 60% of patients.[21]

In COVID-19 have also been described cases of typical and atypical Takotsubo syndrome,[22] possibly triggered by emotional stress and physical stress by infection itself, with a significant increase in the incidence of stress cardiomyopathy when compared with prepandemic periods[23]: echocardiography has a diagnostic role in detecting the typical apical ballooning and possible unfavorable findings (LV outflow tract obstruction, mitral regurgitation, apical thrombus).[24]

Of particular interest, is COVID-19-related myocarditis: a direct cardiotropic localization of

a Cardiology Unit, Luigi Sacco University Hospital, Milan, Italy; b Division of Cardiology, Johns Hopkins University, Baltimore, MD, USA
* Corresponding author. Department of Cardiology, University Hospital Luigi Sacco, Milan, Italy.
E-mail address: barosi.alberto@asst-fbf-sacco.it

Card Electrophysiol Clin 14 (2022) 71–78
https://doi.org/10.1016/j.ccep.2021.10.007
1877-9182/22/© 2021 Elsevier Inc. All rights reserved.

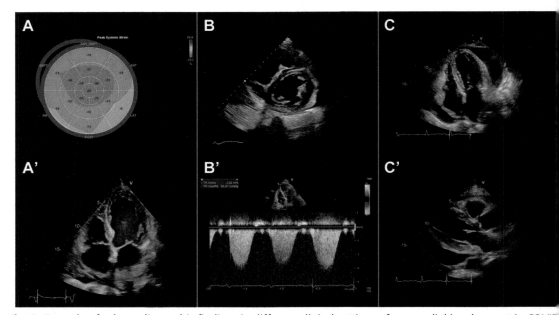

Fig. 1. Example of echocardiographic findings in different clinical settings of myocardial involvement in COVID 19 patients. Panel A and A′: Reduced regional myocardial strain in lateral wall and dilation of left ventricle i myocarditis; Panel B and B′: D-shape of left ventricle and increase in tricuspid regurgitation jet velocity in pulmo nary embolism; Panel C and C′: pericardial effusion, in parasternal long-axis and four-chamber view.

SARS-CoV-2 into myocytes has never been described, but some autoptic findings (lymphocyte infiltrates and macrophagic response) resulted compatible with viral myocarditis.[25] In a systematic review of Sawalha and colleagues comprising 14 cases with myocarditis/myoper carditis believed to have occurred secondary t COVID-19 infection, echocardiography was pe formed in most cases (83%) and 60% had reduce LVEF, with diffuse hypokinesis in 30% o patients.[26]

However, excluding specific clinical scenari while big alterations at conventional echocardiog raphy could be difficult to detect,[27] deformatio imaging can be the appropriate tool to identif subclinical modifications[28]: in a study of Stob and colleagues, despite normal LVEF, most o the infected patients (that ranged from mild to se vere symptoms) showed abnormal LV deforma tion, in particular a reduced longitudinal strai observed predominantly in more than one bas LV segment (in 10/14 patients, 71%), that wa attributed to a possible subepimyocardial involve ment of SARS-CoV-2–induced myocarditi confirmed by cardiac magnetic resonance (CMF but only in 2 patients.[29] Left ventricular-global lor gitudinal strain (LV-GLS) was altered in up to 80% of patients hospitalized for COVID-19 infection[3] (32/40 patients, mean LV-GLS of 12.1% ± 4.0 normal <16%) and was superior to LVEF for pre dicting adverse outcome.[31] Indeed, an importar role of echocardiography could be the prognosti stratification of patients: LV-GLS was found to b an independent predictor of mortality throug multivariate analysis.[32–34]

Table 1 Characteristics echocardiographic findings in different clinical settings of myocardial involvement in COVID-19 patients	
Myocarditis	• LV dilation • LV pseudohypertrophy • LV diffuse hypokinesis • Reduction in LVEF
Acute coronary syndromes	• Regional LV wall-motion abnormalities • Mechanical complications
Pulmonary embolism	• RV dilation with D-shape of LV • RV dysfunction • McConnell's sign • Increase in sPAP
Pericarditis	• Pericardial effusion, possible cardiac tamponade • Brightness of pericardium

Abbreviations: LV, left ventricle; LVEF, left ventricular ejection fraction; RV, right ventricle; sPAP, systolic pulmonary arterial pressure.

A major role in COVID-19 is played by the right ventricle (RV): it could be affected secondarily to elevation in RV afterload; increases in PVR causes RV dilation and eventual RV failure, which has been related to a worse prognosis.[35]

COVID-19 could cause acute respiratory distress syndrome (ARDS) through vasoactive mediators, vascular thrombosis, and vascular compression secondary to atelectasis and edema.[36]

Moreover, patients with COVID-19 are in a prothrombotic state that predisposes them to thromboembolic events, including deep vein thrombosis and pulmonary embolism (PE).[37–39]

The study by Dweck and colleagues, a survey of the European Association of Cardiovascular Imaging, found that 33% of patients had an abnormal RV on echocardiography.[40] Of these subjects, 9% had mild-to-moderate RV dysfunction and % had severe dysfunction (of note, the index used for the definition of dysfunction was not specified). The RV was dilated in 15%, a D-shaped RV was seen in 4% and pulmonary artery pressure was elevated in 8%.

In the study by Mahmoud-Elsayed and colleagues, 41% of patients had a dilated RV (RV basal diameter >41 mm) and 27% had a decreased RV function (fractional area change 35% or a tricuspid annular plane systolic excursion <17 mm); most patients had severe respiratory failure and 82% were on invasive mechanical ventilation. A PE was detected in 0% of subjects with RV dysfunction as compared with 2% in those without RV dysfunction.[41]

Jain and colleagues found that 15.3% of the patients had an increased RV size (12.5% were mildly increased and 2.8% were moderately increased).[42] RV systolic function (assessed semi-quantitatively) was mildly decreased in 26.4%, moderately decreased in 9.7%, and severely decreased in 4.2%.

Several studies reported an association between right-side TTE parameters and prognosis in patients with COVID-19.

Kim and colleagues in an analysis from a US multicentre retrospective study reported that adverse RV remodeling (dysfunction/dilation) conferred a >2 fold increase in mortality risk.[43]

Szekely and colleagues[44] found that the most frequent abnormality among patients with clinical deterioration during follow-up was RV dilatation (with or without dysfunction). In univariable analysis, they reported that shorter pulmonary acceleration time (<100 msec) was associated with clinical deterioration and that RV end-diastolic area was associated with mortality.[44]

Li and colleagues reported that RV global longitudinal strain was a powerful predictor of death in patients with COVID-19.[45]

In a recent systematic review, Messina and colleagues analyzed studies available in literature and concluded that they have highly variable sample sizes and reported highly heterogeneous findings: LVEF does not seem significantly affected (reported as higher than 50% in most subjects), LV diastolic function has not been properly assessed and RV dysfunction seems frequent but defined with variable criteria, making it difficult to establish a clear association with higher mortality.[46]

CARDIAC VALVES AND PERICARDIUM

The presence of valvular heart disease (VHD) has been described in COVID-19 patients undergoing echocardiography during the hospital stay.[40] These valvular diseases more likely were present before the onset of SARS-CoV-2 infection. A recent study regarding echocardiographic findings among COVID patients reported that half of them presented a significant tricuspid regurgitation followed by aortic regurgitation and mitral regurgitation.[47] Tricuspid regurgitation is the most common VHD reported in COVID-19 patients and its severity could directly reflect the impairment of the pulmonary circulation during the infection resulting in pulmonary hypertension, especially in patients with severe pneumonia and respiratory insufficiency.[48]

A higher concern, especially in COVID-19 patients in the intensive care unit, is the presence of infectious endocarditis (IE). Some clinical reports have reported endocarditis in a minority prevalence and the presence of valve vegetations were also described in autopsy findings for SARS-CoV-2 patients.[40,49] In this setting, endocarditis is related to bacterial endocarditis or the presence of thrombus; less likely could be caused by the direct SARS-CoV-2 infection and there is no evidence about that relationship.

According to the American Society of Echocardiography (ASE) and the European Association of Cardiovascular Imaging (EACVI) recommendations, in case of suspected or confirmed SARS-CoV-2 infections, cardiac imaging should be considered only on an individual basis when it could change the clinical management or be lifesaving for the patients, because of the higher risk of contamination for health care providers, especially during transesophageal echocardiography (TOE).[50,51] Despite that, TOE remains the gold standard for the diagnosis of IE even in the current COVID-19 pandemic and to better evaluate the severity of a significant VHD.[52,53] In conclusion, in COVID-19 patients with high suspicion of IE or significant VHD, explorative TTE and if inconclusive a subsequent TOE is mandatory for the diagnosis with all the precautions aimed at avoiding the spread of the infectious disease.

Some case reports reported acute pericarditis during SARS-COV-2 infection.[54] This type of cardiac involvement is often seen in patients with troponin elevation in the context of myocardial damage and less frequently as a primary presentation of COVID-19 infection, which occurred most in younger patients.[55,56] Pericardial involvement may be driven by the systemic and local inflammatory response to infection and less likely by direct virus damage.[57] Another form of pericardial involvement is pericardial effusion, found in nearly 5% of COVID-19 patients who underwent chest CT.

As recommended by ESC guidelines, also in patients with SARS-CoV-2 infection, TTE is recommended as the first diagnostic tool to evaluate pericardial diseases and it is most useful to address the severity of significant effusion.[58] As second step, in selected cases because of logistic issues in this setting, CMR can evaluate pericardial thickening or small effusions, assess myocardial damage, and precisely define pericardial inflammation.[59]

PRACTICAL ASPECTS

Since the beginning of the pandemic, concerns have been raised about the risk of performing echocardiograms for the risk of personnel infection, with the subsequent need to select patients in which echocardiography can have a fundamental diagnostic/prognostic role. The principal echocardiography societies released recommendations to review the appropriateness of every examination, favor the use of handheld devices (easier to disinfect) and perform fast and focused evaluations: they provided a modified point-of-care ultrasound (POCUS) protocol for the evaluation of patients with suspected or confirmed COVID-19, when is likely to have an impact on patient management (summary recommendations in **Box 1**).[50,60] Adopting protocols aimed at reducing the number of inappropriate studies, the workflow in echocardiography laboratories has declined by 50% and the study appropriateness has significantly increased.[61] Moreover, the use of limited tablet-based echocardiograms can reduce the study time by 79%.[62] Considering the importance of prone position in patients developing ARDS, some reports have suggested that prone position echocardiography might be feasible, allowing RV and LV evaluation in a four-chamber view.[63]

Box 1
Summary recommendations for echocardiography in COVID-19 patients

Indications
- Perform urgent/emergent examinations (that can change patient management or be life-saving, in particular for TOE)
- Defer elective/routine follow-up examinations

Personnel protection
- Droplet precautions for TTE (protective clothing, gloves, headcovers, specific face-masks, and eye shields)
- Airborne precautions for TOE (N-95 or N-99 respirator masks)
- Patients should wear a surgical mask during imaging

Method
- Focus cardiac ultrasound study:

     LV: LVEF, regional dysfunction, end-diastolic cavity dimension

     RV: TAPSE, end-diastolic cavity dimension, tricuspid regurgitation pressure gradient

     Valves: gross signs of valvular disease

     Pericardium: thickening or effusion
- ECG monitoring can be omitted

Technology
- Prefer hand-held or smaller lap-top–based scanners
- Measurements should be performed offline

Abbreviations: LV, left ventricle; LVEF, left ventricular ejection fraction; RV, right ventricle; TAPSE, tricuspid annular plane systolic excursion; TOE, transesophageal echocardiography; TTE, transthoracic echocardiography.

DEVELOPMENT OF NEW TECHNOLOGIES

The need for absolute isolation of symptomatic patients and the high possibility of spreading the infection outside the isolation rooms in the high intensity care departments, makes any attempt a an instrumental diagnostic approach difficult, give also the absolute need to decontaminate the equipment used after each individual examination. Th advantages deriving from the execution of echocardiography examination at the patient's bedside a well known but the high risk of serious coronavirus infection diffusion has made its use difficult. Disinfection is the only way to counter the risk spreading the disease from one patient to another r among the operators themselves, which event is even more dangerous because it would jeopardize the tightness of the system. Hand-carried echocardiography devices offer rapid and readily available information at the bedside, as they help overcome the problems caused by the use of cumbersome standard equipment.[62,64] The use of "ultramobile devices" has recently been introduced in the area of cardiovascular ultrasound diagnostics. These devices are miniaturized systems equipped with diagnostic quality two-dimensional (2D) and color Doppler imaging. With simplified criteria, they can detect LV dysfunction and moderate-severe valvulopathy with good sensitivity and specificity. They are extremely useful in the immediate diagnosis of pericardial effusion and in the definition of states of cardiocirculatory failure or inflammatory states of pulmonary parenchyma. In resource-limited settings, ultramobile systems can reduce the need for standard echocardiography. "Ultramobile" systems have a probe that can be connected to any handheld device, smartphone, or tablet, allowing the execution of cardiac, pulmonary, vascular, abdominal, soft tissue, and joint ultrasound. The isolation system, required to avoid the danger of spreading the infection, is simple, consisting of a mono-use coating sheath commonly used for epicardial echocardiography in the cardiac surgery operating room. At the end of the examination, the probe is removed from the casing, reinserted in a new protective sheath, and ready for a subsequent examination. The compactness of the system makes it easily isolable from the environment with a mono-use coating sheath, making it very practical in environments with a high level of contamination or where absolute sterility is required. Thanks to internet connectivity, the images, stored in DICOM format, can also be simultaneously viewed in real time by other doctors outside the contaminated area: data collection and their quick transfer allow postprocedural analysis in the safe zone. Finally, a video call system allows communication between operators. Moreover, this aspect gives the possibility to exploit few medical imaging experts for the interpretation of examinations from numerous Spot Centers, also performed by doctors or trained nonmedical staff not specialized in imaging.

Moreover, in China, a pilot study of robot-assisted teleultrasound based on 5G Network was conducted[65]: ultrasound specialists carried out the robot-assisted teleultrasound, manipulating a handheld controller, which can control the robotic arm, and did remote consultation in order to settle the problem of early cardiopulmonary evaluation in COVID-19 patients.

A point of particular importance is the role of artificial intelligence (AI), technology that creates a computerized model to solve different problems without the requirement of human assistance, continuously learns from the data set, and predicts outcomes accurately.[66,67] It was used in intensive care unit by critical care physicians without formal training in ultrasound to obtain POCUS images, with the use of real-time prescriptive guidance to direct the physician's transducer position and hand movements to acquire the images, automatically capturing them when appropriate, detecting LVEF with high accuracy, and uploading to the archive and communication system for offline review.[68] AI includes machine learning (ML), which offers the potential to improve the accuracy and reliability of echocardiography by combining clinician interpretation with information derived from ML algorithms. In conclusion, high volume data generated from cardiac imaging can be integrated into a multiparametric approach for pattern recognition and imaging data-based disease phenotype characterization, particularly useful and time-saving in the setting on COVID-19 pandemic.[69]

SUMMARY

Echocardiography has a diagnostic and prognostic role in COVID-19, helping in recognizing cardiac involvement. Considering the high risk of personnel infection and equipment contamination, focused echocardiographic protocols with portable devices are recommended.

Available echocardiographic data on COVID-19 patients actually do not provide definite evidence, due to multiple factors: high heterogeneity between studies in numbers of patients, miscellaneous results, and low quality of echocardiographic studies for technical difficulties in performing bedside procedures (patients with respiratory distress/invasive ventilation; while wearing personal protective equipment).

In conclusion, echocardiography represents an important tool in the management of COVID-19 patients, but more studies with standardized acquisitions and methods are needed to describe definite echocardiographic findings in this setting.

CLINICS CARE POINTS

- Focused echocardiographic protocols can detect cardiac involvement in COVID-19
- Echocardiography is strictly recommended if it could change the clinical management

• Available data do not provide definite evidence on echocardiographic findings in COVID-19

REFERENCES

1. Busana M, Gasperetti A, Giosa L, et al. Prevalence and outcome of silent hypoxemia in COVID-19. Minerva Anestesiol 2021;87(3):325–33.
2. Zheng YY, Ma YT, Zhang JY, et al. COVID-19 and the cardiovascular system. Nat Rev Cardiol 2020;17(5):259–60.
3. Kang Y, Chen T, Mui D, et al. Cardiovascular manifestations and treatment considerations in COVID-19. Heart 2020;106(15):1132–41.
4. Shi S, Qin M, Shen B, et al. Association of cardiac injury with mortality in hospitalized patients with COVID-19 in Wuhan, China. JAMA Cardiol 2020;5(7):802–10.
5. De Filippo O, D'Ascenzo F, Angelini F, et al. Reduced rate of hospital admissions for ACS during covid-19 outbreak in Northern Italy. N Engl J Med 2020;383(1):88–9.
6. Severino P, D'Amato A, Saglietto A, et al. Reduction in heart failure hospitalization rate during coronavirus disease 19 pandemic outbreak. ESC Hear Fail 2020;7(6):4182–8.
7. De Rosa S, Spaccarotella C, Basso C, et al. Reduction of hospitalizations for myocardial infarction in Italy in the COVID-19 era. Eur Heart J 2020;41(22):2083–8.
8. Schiavone M, Forleo GB, Mitacchione G, et al. Quis custodiet ipsos custodes: are we taking care of healthcare workers in the Italian COVID-19 outbreak? J Hosp Infect 2020;105(3):580–1.
9. Capaccione KM, Leb JS, Belinda D, et al. Acute myocardial infarction secondary to COVID-19 infection: a case report and review of the literature. Clin Imaging 2021;72:178–82.
10. Schiavone M, Gobbi C, Biondi-Zoccai G, et al. Acute coronary syndromes and covid-19: exploring the uncertainties. J Clin Med 2020;9(6):1683.
11. Schiavone M, Gasperetti A, Mancone M, et al. Redefining the prognostic value of high-sensitivity troponin in COVID-19 patients: the importance of concomitant coronary artery disease. J Clin Med 2020;9(10):3263.
12. Gomez JMD, Nair G, Nanavaty P, et al. COVID-19-associated takotsubo cardiomyopathy. BMJ Case Rep 2020;13(12):1–5.
13. Zeng JH, Liu YX, Yuan J, et al. First case of COVID-19 complicated with fulminant myocarditis: a case report and insights. Infection 2020;48(5):773–7.
14. Mitacchione G, Schiavone M, Gasperetti A, et al. Ventricular tachycardia storm management in a COVID-19 patient: a case report. Eur Heart J Case Rep 2020;4(FI1):1–6.
15. Schiavone M, Gasperetti A, Mancone M, et al. Oral anticoagulation and clinical outcomes in COVID-19: an Italian multicenter experience. Int J Cardiol 2021;323:276–80.
16. Gasperetti A, Biffi M, Duru F, et al. Arrhythmic safety of hydroxychloroquine in COVID-19 patients from different clinical settings. Europace 2020;22(12):1855–63.
17. Chang WT, Toh HS, Liao C Te, et al. Cardiac involvement of COVID-19: a comprehensive review. Am J Med Sci 2021;361(1):14–22.
18. Mitacchione G, Schiavone M, Curnis A, et al. Impact of prior statin use on clinical outcomes in COVID-19 patients: data from tertiary referral hospitals during COVID-19 pandemic in Italy. J Clin Lipidol 2021;15(1):68–78.
19. Guo T, Fan Y, Chen M, et al. Cardiovascular implications of fatal outcomes of patients with coronavirus disease 2019 (COVID-19). JAMA Cardiol 2020;5(7):811–8.
20. Bergamaschi L, D'Angelo EC, Paolisso P, et al. The value of ECG changes in risk stratification of COVID-19 patients. Ann Noninvasive Electrocardiol 2021;26(3):1–10.
21. Stefanini GG, Montorfano M, Trabattoni D, et al. ST elevation myocardial infarction in patients with COVID-19: clinical and angiographic outcomes. Circulation 2020;2113–6. https://doi.org/10.116 CIRCULATIONAHA.120.047525.
22. Meyer P, Degrauwe S, Van Delden C, et al. Typical takotsubo syndrome triggered by SARS-CoV-infection. Eur Heart J 2020;41(19):1860.
23. Jabri A, Kalra A, Reed GW. Incidence of stress cardiomyopathy during the coronavirus disease 2019 pandemic main outcomes and measures. JAMA Netw Open 2020;3(7):e2014780.
24. Okura H. Update of takotsubo syndrome in the era of COVID-19. J Cardiol 2021;77:361–9.
25. Tavazzi G, Pellegrini C, Maurelli M, et al. Myocardial localization of coronavirus in COVID-19 cardiogenic shock. Eur J Heart Fail 2020;22(5):911–5.
26. Sawalha K, Abozenah M, Kadado AJ, et al. Systematic review of COVID-19 related myocarditis: insights on management and outcome. Cardiovasc Revasc Med 2021;23(xxxx):107–13.
27. Ceriani E, Marceca A, Lanfranchi A, et al. Early echocardiographic findings in patients hospitalized for COVID-19 pneumonia: a prospective, single center study. Intern Emerg Med 2021;(0123456789) https://doi.org/10.1007/s11739-021-02733-9.
28. Busana M, Schiavone M, Lanfranchi A, et al. Noninvasive hemodynamic profile of early COVID-19 infection. Physiol Rep 2020;8(20). https://doi.org 10.14814/phy2.14628.
29. Stöbe S, Richter S, Seige M, et al. Echocardiographic characteristics of patients with SARS - CoV - 2 infection. Clin Res Cardiol 2020;109(12):1549–66.

0. Shmueli H, Shah M, Ebinger JE, et al. Left ventricular global longitudinal strain in identifying subclinical myocardial dysfunction among patients hospitalized with COVID-19. IJC Hear Vasc 2021;32:100719.

1. Rothschild E, Baruch G, Szekely Y, et al. The predictive role of left and right ventricular speckle-tracking echocardiography in COVID-19. JACC Cardiovasc Imaging 2020;13(11):2471–4.

2. Faruk O, Hasan B, Barman A, et al. Evaluation of biventricular function in patients with COVID - 19 using speckle tracking echocardiography. Int J Cardiovasc Imaging 2020;(0123456789). https://doi.org/10.1007/s10554-020-01968-5.

3. Janus SE, Hajjari J, Karnib M, et al. Prognostic value of left ventricular global longitudinal strain in COVID-19. Am J Cardiol 2020;131:134–6.

4. Wibowo A, Pranata R, Astuti A, et al. Left and right ventricular longitudinal strains are associated with poor outcome in COVID-19: a systematic review and meta- analysis. J Intensive Care 2021;9:9.

5. Berlin DA, Gulick RM, Martinez FJ. Severe covid-19. N Engl J Med 2020;383(25):2451–60.

6. Park JF, Banerjee S, Umar S. In the eye of the storm: the right ventricle in COVID-19. Pulm Circ 2020; 10(3).

7. Nishiga M, Wang DW, Han Y, et al. COVID-19 and cardiovascular disease: from basic mechanisms to clinical perspectives. Nat Rev Cardiol 2020;17(9): 543–58.

8. Danzi GB, Loffi M, Galeazzi G, et al. Acute pulmonary embolism and COVID-19 pneumonia: a random association? Eur Heart J 2020;41(19). https://doi.org/10.1093/eurheartj/ehaa254.

9. Paolisso P, Bergamaschi L, D'Angelo EC, et al. Preliminary experience with low molecular Weight Heparin Strategy in COVID-19 patients. Front Pharmacol 2020;11:1–6.

0. Dweck MR, Bularga A, Hahn RT, et al. Global evaluation of echocardiography in patients with COVID-19. Eur Heart J Cardiovasc Imaging 2020;21(9): 949–58.

1. Mahmoud-Elsayed HM, Moody WE, Bradlow WM, et al. Echocardiographic findings in patients with COVID-19 pneumonia. Can J Cardiol 2020;36(8): 1203–7.

2. Jain SS, Liu Q, Raikhelkar J, et al. Indications for and findings on transthoracic echocardiography in COVID-19. J Am Soc Echocardiogr 2020;33(10): 1278–84.

3. Kim J, Volodarskiy A, Sultana R, et al. Prognostic utility of right ventricular remodeling over conventional risk stratification in patients with COVID-19. J Am Coll Cardiol 2020;(17):1965–77.

4. Szekely Y, Lichter Y, Taieb P, et al. Spectrum of cardiac manifestations in COVID-19: a systematic echocardiographic study. Circulation 2020;142(4): 342–53.

45. Li Y, Li H, Zhu S, et al. Prognostic value of right ventricular longitudinal strain in patients with COVID-19. JACC Cardiovasc Imaging 2020;13(11):2287–99.

46. Messina A, Sanfilippo F, Milani A, et al. COVID-19-related echocardiographic patterns of cardiovascular dysfunction in critically ill patients: a systematic review of the current literature. J Crit Care 2021;65: 26–35.

47. Khan A, James S, Yuan M, Woolery L, Huppertz N. Observations on echocardiographic ndings in patients with COVID-19. Preprint from Research Square. https://doi.org/10.21203/rs.3.rs-58076/v1.

48. Carrizales-Sepúlveda EF, Vera-Pineda R, Flores-Ramírez R, et al. Echocardiographic manifestations in COVID-19: a review. Hear Lung Circ 2021. https://doi.org/10.1016/j.hlc.2021.02.004.

49. Chong PY, Chui P, Ling AE, et al. Analysis of deaths during the severe acute respiratory syndrome (SARS) epidemic in Singapore: challenges in Determining a SARS diagnosis. Arch Pathol Lab Med 2004;128(2):195–204.

50. Skulstad H, Cosyns B, Popescu BA, et al. COVID-19 pandemic and cardiac imaging: EACVI recommendations on precautions, indications, prioritization, and protection for patients and healthcare personnel. Eur Heart J Cardiovasc Imaging 2020; 21(6):592–8.

51. Kirkpatrick JN, Mitchell C, Taub C, et al. ASE Statement on protection of patients and echocardiography Service providers during the 2019 Novel coronavirus outbreak: endorsed by the American college of cardiology. J Am Soc Echocardiogr 2020;33(6):648–53.

52. Habib G, Lancellotti P, Antunes MJ, et al. 2015 ESC guidelines for the management of infective endocarditis. Eur Heart J 2015;36(44):3036–7.

53. Baumgartner H, Falk V, Bax JJ, et al. 2017 ESC/EACTS guidelines for the management of valvular heart disease. Eur Heart J 2017;38(36):2739–91.

54. Furqan MM, Verma BR, Cremer PC, et al. Pericardial diseases in COVID19: a contemporary review. Curr Cardiol Rep 2021;23(7). https://doi.org/10.1007/s11886-021-01519-x.

55. Kumar R, Kumar J, Daly C, et al. Acute pericarditis as a primary presentation of COVID-19. BMJ Case Rep 2020;13(8):1–3.

56. Dimopoulou D, Spyridis N, Dasoula F, et al. Pericarditis as the main clinical manifestation of covid-19 in adolescents. Pediatr Infect Dis J 2021;40(5):E197–9.

57. Manjili RH, Zarei M, Habibi M, et al. COVID-19 as an acute inflammatory disease. J Immunol 2020;205(1): 12–9.

58. Adler Y, Charron P, Imazio M, et al. 2015 ESC Guidelines for the diagnosis and management of pericardial diseases. Eur Heart J 2015;36(42):2921–64.

59. Imazio M, Brucato A, Lazaros G, et al. Anti-inflammatory therapies for pericardial diseases in the

COVID-19 pandemic: safety and potentiality. J Cardiovasc Med (Hagerstown) 2020;21(9):625–9.

60. Christian M, Lassen H, Skaarup KG, et al. Echocardiographic abnormalities and predictors of mortality in hospitalized COVID - 19 patients : the ECHOVID - 19 study. ESC Heart Fail 2020;7(6):4189–97.

61. Ward RP, Lee L, Ward TJ, et al. Utilization and appropriateness of transthoracic echocardiography in response to the COVID-19 pandemic. J Am Soc Echocardiogr 2020;33(6):690–1.

62. McMahon SR, De Francis G, Schwartz S, et al. Tablet-based limited echocardiography to reduce Sonographer scan and decontamination time during the COVID-19 pandemic. J Am Soc Echocardiogr 2020;33(7):895–9.

63. García-Cruz E, Manzur-Sandoval D, Gopar-Nieto R, et al. Transthoracic echocardiography during prone position ventilation: Lessons from the COVID-19 pandemic. J Am Coll Emerg Physicians Open 2020;1(5):730–6.

64. Elikowski W, Malek-Elikowska M, Fertala N, et al. Tablet-based limited echocardiography at COVID-19-dedicated hospital during the pandemic in the context of takotsubo syndrome. Pol Merkur Lekarski 2021;49(289):57–9.

65. Wu S, Wu D, Ye R, et al. Pilot study of robot-assisted teleultrasound based on 5G Network: a new feasible Strategy for early imaging Assessment during COVID-19 pandemic. IEEE Trans Ultrason Ferroelectr Freq Control 2020;67(11):2241–8.

66. Kagiyama N, Shrestha S, Farjo PD, et al. Artificial intelligence: practical primer for clinical Research cardiovascular disease. J Am Heart Assoc 2019 8(17):e012788.

67. Bitetto A, Bianchi E, Dondi P, et al. Deep learning detection of cardiac Akinesis in echocardiograms, vol 12661 LNCS. Springer International Publishing; 2021. p. 503–14. Available at: https://search.bvsalud.org/global-literature-on-novel-coronavirus-2019-ncov/resource/es/covidwho-1198421.

68. Cheema BS, Walter J, Narang A, et al. Artificial intelligence–enabled POCUS in the COVID-19 ICU: a new Spin on cardiac ultrasound. JACC Case Rep 2021;3(2):258–63.

69. Zimmerman A, Kalra D. Usefulness of machine learning in COVID-19 for the detection and prognosis of cardiovascular complications. Rev Cardiovasc Med 2020;21(3):345–52.

Imaging Findings of COVID-19–Related Cardiovascular Complications

Eleni Nakou, MD, PhD[a], Estefania De Garate, MD[b], Kate Liang, MBBCh[b], Matthew Williams, MBChB, BSc[b], Dudley J. Pennell, MD[c], Chiara Bucciarelli-Ducci, MD, PhD[d],*

KEYWORDS

- COVID-19 • Myocardial injury • Cardiovascular magnetic resonance (CMR) • Myocarditis
- Pulmonary embolism

KEY POINTS

- Cardiovascular manifestations are common in COVID-19 patients with prognostic implications.
- Most COVID-19–related cardiovascular complications are mainly the consequences of myocardial injury, although the pathophysiological mechanisms are still under investigation.
- Common COVID-19-related cardiovascular manifestations include acute coronary syndromes, myo/pericarditis, pulmonary embolism, and heart failure.
- Advanced cardiac imaging plays an essential role in the diagnosis of cardiac complications and the risk stratification of COVID-19 patients.

INTRODUCTION

At the end of 2019, the severe acute respiratory syndrome coronavirus 2 (SARS-CoV-2) was identified as a novel cause of respiratory infection in Wuhan, which spread rapidly resulting in the global pandemic of coronavirus disease (COVID-19).[1] It is widely recognized that patients with cardiovascular (CV) risk factors, or established CV disease (CVD), are at increased risk of developing severe COVID-19, and those with myocardial injury have a worse prognosis.[2–5] Studies have shown that COVID-19 can cause a broad spectrum of CV complications including myocarditis,[6] myocardial infarction (MI),[7] stress cardiomyopathy,[8] heart failure (HF),[9] arrhythmias,[10] thromboembolic events,[11] and cardiogenic shock.[12] Advanced cardiac imaging is a reliable diagnostic

tool for prompt diagnosis, risk stratification, monitoring, and management of patients with COVID-19–related CV manifestations. This review is focused on the role of multimodality imaging in identifying cardiac involvement in COVID-19 and the potential CV side effects of the available treatment and vaccines against SARS-CoV-2.

PATHOGENESIS OF COVID-19–ASSOCIATED CV COMPLICATIONS

Although the pathophysiological mechanisms of the myocardial injury caused by SARS-CoV-2 have not been entirely elucidated, multiple factors have been hypothesized to contribute directly or indirectly to the development of CV complications.

a. *Direct virus-mediated cytotoxicity.* Although this theory is supported by an autopsy series,

[a] CMR Unit, Royal Brompton and Harefield Hospitals, Guys and St Thomas NHS Foundation Trust, Sydney Street, London, SW3 6NP, UK; [b] Bristol Heart Institute, University Hospitals Bristol and Weston NHS Trust and University of Bristol, Upper Maudlin St, Bristol, BS2 8HW, UK; [c] Royal Brompton and Harefield Hospitals, Guys and St Thomas NHS Trust and Imperial College London, London, SW3 6NP, UK; [d] Royal Brompton and Harefield Hospitals, Guys and St Thomas NHS Trust and King's College London, Sydney Street, London, SW3 6NP, UK
* Corresponding author. Royal Brompton Hospital, Sydney Street, London, SW3 6NP, United Kingdom
E-mail address: c.bucciarelli-ducci@rbht.nhs.uk

Card Electrophysiol Clin 14 (2022) 79–93
https://doi.org/10.1016/j.ccep.2021.10.008

which confirmed the detection of viral genome detection within the myocardium,[13,14] in clinical practice, the histologic evidence of myocardial injury in COVID-19 is limited. Low loads of viral genome were detected in histology specimens in 5 cases out of 104 patients undergoing endomyocardial biopsy (EMB) for myocarditis or unexplained HF during the COVID-19 pandemic.[15] However, there was no evidence of myocardial injury detected in the autopsy of a patient with COVID-19 and acute respiratory distress syndrome, who died of sudden cardiac death, challenging the theory of a direct cardiotoxic effect of SARS-CoV-2.[16]

b. *Dysregulation of renin-angiotensin-aldosterone system.* There is evidence that SARS-CoV-2 infection might cause downregulation of angiotensin-converting enzyme 2 (ACE2),[17] which has a cardioprotective role as an antifibrotic, antioxidating, and anti-inflammatory factor.[17] In addition, the connection of the viral protein S to human ACE2 can downregulate the degradation of angiotensin 2 to angiotensin 1-7.[18] The accumulation of angiotensin 2 might activate the p38 Mitogen-Activated Protein Kinase (MAPK) pathway promoting thrombotic events[19] and might also induce the production of reactive oxygen species (ROS) causing myocardial injury.[20]

c. *Endothelial cell damage and thromboinflammation.* The direct invasion of the vascular endothelial cells via ACE2 receptors may result in inflammation and endothelial dysfunction contributing to thrombosis. There is early histologic evidence of direct toxic effects to endothelial cells caused by SARS-CoV-2.[21] In this case series, there was evidence of lymphocytic endotheliitis in the lungs, heart, and kidneys in a patient who died from COVID-19 and multiorgan failure. This was also observed in the lungs, heart, kidneys, and liver in a patient who died with COVID-19, multisystem inflammatory response (MIS), and MI with ST elevation.

d. *Dysregulation of immune response.* It is hypothesized that the SARS-CoV-2 infection can induce an excessive activation of immune cells and inflammatory response causing a cytokine storm. The overproduction of proinflammatory cytokines can lead to endothelial dysfunction and the activation of complement pathways, platelets, von Willebrand factor, and tissue factor; increasing the risk of thrombosis in the circulation including in the coronary system, and therefore increasing the risk of an acute coronary syndrome.[22,23] SARS-CoV-2 infection can also promote a disproportionate production of factor VIII and neutrophil extracellular traps, which can facilitate the development of thrombotic events.[22–24] Apart from type I MI, the exaggerated systemic inflammatory response increases the metabolic demand causing myocardial mismatch in oxygen demand and supply and, as a consequence, type II MI.[23–25]

e. *Hypoxic injury.* Hypoxia caused by SARS-CoV-2 infection induces intracellular acidosis and the release of ROS from mitochondria in cardiomyocytes, which destroys the cell membrane contributing to cardiomyocyte apoptosis.[4,26]

f. *Cardiovascular side effects of drugs and vaccines.* It is widely known that antiretroviral therapy and other drugs used in the management of COVID-19 patients (azithromycin, tocilizumab, chloroquine, and hydroxychloroquine) can induce arrhythmias, or interact with some CV treatments.[27] In addition, cases of thromboembolic events have been reported after ChAdOx1 nCov-19/AZD1222 (AstraZeneca COVID-19 vaccine) and Ad26.COV2.S (Janssen COVID-19 vaccine)[28,29] vaccinations. More recently, there is a potential association of the mRNA vaccines, BNTb162b (Pfizer) and mRNA-1273 (Moderna) with myocarditis.[30] is currently believed that the thrombotic events have been associated with autoantibodies directed against the platelet factor 4 (PF4) antigen.[31]

The underlying pathophysiological mechanisms causing COVID-19–related CV complications are presented in **Fig. 1**.

THE ROLE OF IMAGING TECHNIQUES IN DIAGNOSIS, PROGNOSIS, AND MANAGEMENT OF COVID-19–RELATED CV COMPLICATIONS

There is increasing evidence that patients with pre-existing CVD are at an increased risk of developing acute myocardial injury, with high troponin levels associated with a poorer prognosis.[2] Studies show that 12% to 15% of hospitalized COVID-19 patients had an elevated troponin suggestive of myocardial damage, whereas up to 31% with severe COVID-19 presentation had cardiac involvement.[32,33] Another study with 112 patients with COVID-19 showed that troponin levels were mostly normal at admission. Troponin increased during hospitalization in 37.5% of the patients, especially in those who died, whereas typical signs of myocarditis were not detected on echocardiography.[34] These findings suggested that myocardial injury might be the consequence of the systemic inflammatory response rather

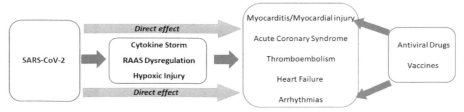

ig. 1. The pathophysiological interaction between cardiovascular system and COVID-19 showing the potential nderlying mechanisms in the development of cardiovascular complications. COVID-19, coronovirus disease 019; RAAS, renin-angiotensin-aldosterone system; SARS-CoV-2, severe acute respiratory syndrome coronavirus 2.

han the direct invasion and damage by SARS-CoV-2.

ransthoracic Echocardiography

n a study of 305 hospitalized patients with COVID 9, myocardial injury (defined by elevated troponin evels) was observed in 190 patients.[35] Echocardiographic abnormalities, including global or egional left ventricular (LV) wall motion abnormalies, LV diastolic dysfunction, right ventricular (RV) ysfunction, and pericardial effusions were noted n almost two-thirds of patients with myocardial njury. In the same study, the detection of structural abnormalities by transthoracic echocardiography (TTE) was an independent predictive factor f mortality in the subgroup with myocardial injury. n international prospective study of 1216 patients om 69 countries with clinical indication for TTE evealed the spectrum of echocardiographic abormalities.[36] Abnormal TTE was found in 55%, ncluding LV and RV abnormalities at 39% and 3% respectively, whereas the prevalence of chocardiographic abnormalities was slightly ower (46%) in the subgroup with no pre-existing VD. The LV abnormalities were predominantly onspecific in nature and the mechanism of ysfunction was often not identified unless the TE findings were suggestive of acute MI (3%), yocarditis (3%), and stress cardiomyopathy 2%). In the same study, severe LV, RV, or biven-icular systolic dysfunction was observed in 4% and cardiac tamponade occurred in 1%. In ontrast, another study showed that RV dilatation nd systolic dysfunction were more common 39%) compared with LV systolic dysfunction 0%) in 100 hospitalized patients with COVID-19 7. The most common echocardiographic findings mong those with subsequent clinical deteriora-on were worsening RV and LV function (12 and patients respectively).

Myocardial infarction, myocarditis, or acute pulonary hypertension might be the cause of iso-ated RV dysfunction in COVID-19 patients.[38] cute cor pulmonale precipitated by acute

pulmonary embolism (PE) or adult respiratory distress syndrome has also been reported.[39–41] In addition, the implementation of positive end-expiratory pressure in the respiratory support of critically ill COVID-19 patients can contribute to RV dysfunction.[42] Interestingly, RV dysfunction has been shown to correlate with poor prognosis in COVID-19.[38,42–44]

Cases of pericardial effusion in the context of pericarditis detected on TTE, either in association with myocarditis or as an isolated presentation, along with rare cases of pericardial tamponade in patients with COVID-19 have also been reported.[45–49] Although there are no studies currently investigating the prevalence of pericardial involvement in COVID-19, the diagnosis of pericarditis should be considered in COVID-19 patients presenting with chest pain, ST elevation in the electrocardiogram (ECG), and normal coronary arteries.

Speckle tracking echocardiography is a novel echocardiographic technique. It allows quantification of myocardial deformation, providing early detection of cardiac dysfunction and plays an important prognostic role in HF and patients with end-stage renal disease.[50,51] In addition, impaired LV and RV longitudinal strain are suggestive of early ventricular dysfunction with prognostic value in COVID-19 patients.[44,52] A specific pattern of prominent longitudinal strain reduction of the basal LV segments has been described in COVID-19 patients suggesting that these areas might be vulnerable to myocardial injury during SARS-CoV-2 infection.[53]

Cardiovascular Magnetic Resonance

Cardiovascular magnetic resonance (CMR) imaging is increasingly recognized as an essential tool in the assessment of COVID-19–induced myocardial injury because of the unique capability of CMR for noninvasive tissue characterization. **Fig. 2** shows the specific CMR techniques used for the characterization of tissue damage in clinical practice. Guidelines have been published for safe CMR

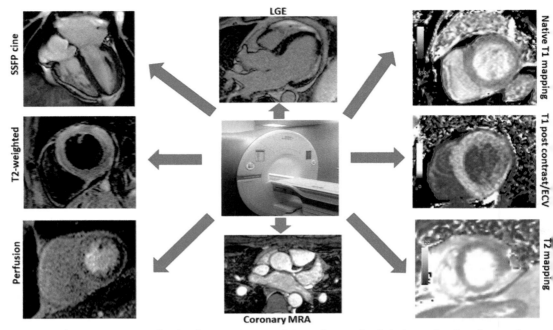

Fig. 2. Specific CMR sequences for the characterization of tissue damage in clinical practice. Steady-state free precession (SSFP) MRI cine: for the assessment of wall motion. T2-weighted imaging: for the assessment of edema. Perfusion imaging: for the assessment of inducible ischemia. Coronary MR angiography (MRA): for the evaluation of the origins of the coronary arteries. Late gadolinium enhancement (LGE): marker of acute myocardial injury, fibrosis, or infarction. Native T1 and T1 postcontrast/extracellular volume (ECV) mapping: for the evaluation of diffuse fibrosis, or infiltration. T2 mapping: a marker of myocardial edema.

scanning during the COVID-19 pandemic[54,55] and the Society for Cardiovascular Magnetic Resonance recommends a specific protocol to perform in patients with suspected COVID-19 cardiac involvement.[56] The primary advantage of CMR is the ability to differentiate between ischemic and nonischemic pathologies.[57] Although EMB remains the gold standard for the diagnosis of acute myocarditis, its use in routine clinical practice is limited because of low diagnostic accuracy and periprocedural risks. The Lake Louise Criteria (LLC) were initially established in 2009 using specific CMR techniques, including T2-weighted sequences, early and late gadolinium enhancement sequences (EGE and LGE, respectively), for the diagnosis of acute myocarditis[58]; expanding them to the use of parametric mapping in the updated version.[59] Therefore, CMR represents a robust noninvasive technique for the diagnosis of COVID-19–related myocarditis. CMR typically shows diffuse myocardial edema, noninfarct patterns of LGE, and increased signal on T2-weighted imaging, T1- and T2-mapping sequences[60] (**Fig. 3**). CMR can also confirm the involvement of pericardium revealing edematous and enhancing pericardial layers suggestive of

pericardial inflammation. Moreover, it has incremental value in differentiating COVID-19–associated stress (Takotsubo) cardiomyopathy and M in patients with SARS-CoV-2 infection presenting with chest pain, high troponin, and ECG abnormalities. The absence of LGE in dysfunctional LV segments with the evidence of edema allows the differentiation from MI when transmural or subendocardial LGE with a coronary distribution is detected (**Fig. 4**).[61] There is also an increased incidence of stress cardiomyopathy in patients without COVID-19 during the pandemic compared with the prepandemic era indicating the intense emotional stress.[62]

CMR abnormalities have been reported in patients who have recently recovered from COVID-19, though most of them have been nonspecific and it is unclear whether they were pre-existing findings and thus unrelated to COVID-19. A study of 100 patients investigated the outcomes of CMR in patients recently recovered from COVID-19, including 18 patients with asymptomatic SARS-CoV-2 infection, 49 patients with mild to moderate symptoms, and 33 patients with severe symptoms requiring hospitalization. Comparisons were made with healthy controls as well as with

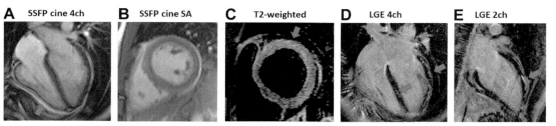

Fig. 3. CMR findings in a 21-year-old COVID-19 patient with acute myopericarditis who presented with chest pain, high troponin levels (1143 ng/L, normal range <14 ng/L), and global mild left ventricular systolic dysfunction on the bedside transthoracic echocardiography (TTE). (*A, B*) Steady-state free precession (SSFP) MRI cine 4 chamber (4ch) and short axis (SA), the arrows show the small pericardial effusion. (*C*) T2-weighted imaging showing slightly increased signal in the basal anterior wall (*arrow*) extending to basal anterolateral wall suggestive of myocardial edema. (*D, E*) Extensive patchy subepicardial and midwall late gadolinium enhancement (LGE) in the basal inferior, midinferoseptal, anterolateral, and anterior walls (*arrows*).

sk factor-matched controls.[63] CMR was performed 2 to 3 months after the initial positive COVID-19 test. Significant high-sensitivity troponin I (hs-cTnI) elevation at the time of CMR was noted in 5% of the patients. Notably, high myocardial native T1 (73%), elevated myocardial native T2 (60%), myocardial LGE (32%), and pericardial LGE (22%) were detected in patients who recovered from COVID-19, whereas CMR abnormalities found in the risk-factor matched controls

were less frequent including high native T1 and T2 (40% and 9%, respectively), myocardial LGE (17%), and pericardial LGE (15%). There was also mild LV and RV systolic dysfunction compared with healthy and risk-factor matched controls (LVEF 56% vs 60% and 61%, respectively; RVEF 56% vs 60% and 59% respectively). Similarly, a smaller study of 26 patients who remained symptomatic after recovery from COVID-19 found myocardial edema in 54%, LGE

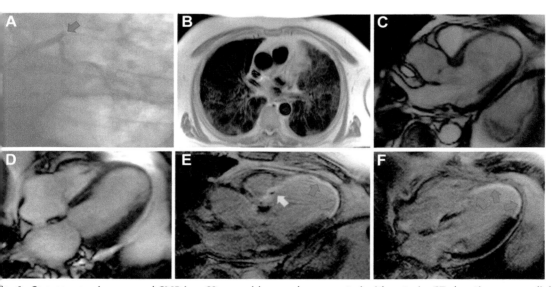

Fig. 4. Coronary angiogram and CMR in a 69-year-old man who presented with anterior ST-elevation myocardial infarction (STEMI) in the context of COVID-19. CMR performed 25 days after the acute coronary syndrome. (*A*) Coronary angiogram showing proximal occlusion (*arrow*) of left anterior descending (LAD) artery with high burden of thrombus. (*B*) CMR axial Half-Fourier Acquisition Single-shot Turbo Spin Echo (HASTE) showing patchy bilateral lung changes of high signal in keeping with COVID-19. (*C, D*) Steady-state free precession (SSFP) MRI cine in endsystole showing thinning and akinesia of mid to apical septal walls extending to apical lateral walls and apical cap. (*E, F*) Late gadolinium enhancement (LGE) imaging showing transmural LGE in the mid to apical septal walls extending to the apical lateral walls and apical cap (*blue arrows*). In addition, there is partial extension of enhancement into the basal septal segments with evidence of microvascular obstruction in the basal anteroseptum (*yellow arrow*).

31%, and decreased RV functional parameters in the subgroup with positive conventional CMR findings.[64] A larger study included 148 patients with severe COVID-19 [all requiring hospital admission, 48 of whom (32%) requiring ventilatory support] and troponin elevation who underwent CMR at a median of 68 days after discharge.[65] LV function was normal in 89%, myocarditis-like scar noted in 26%, infarction and/or ischemia in 22%, and dual pathology in 6%. However, whether these abnormalities represent de novo COVID-19–associated changes or pre-existed in the context of clinically silent disease remains unclear. Importantly, the extent of these abnormalities was quite limited and with minimal functional consequences.

CMR findings have also been reported among athletes who have recovered from COVID-19.[66–68] In a study of 145 university student-athletes who were asymptomatic or experienced mild to moderate symptoms, CMR was performed at a median of 15 days after the positive COVID-19 tests.[67] CMR findings consistent with updated LLC for myocarditis were found in only 2 patients (1.4%), whereas 40 patients (27.6%) had small nonspecific foci of LGE. A smaller study of 26 competitive collegiate athletes who underwent CMR examination 11 to 53 days after diagnosis of COVID-19 showed that 4 athletes (15%) met the updated LLC for clinically suspected myocarditis and 8 athletes (30%) had nonspecific LGE.[66] In the same study, none of the athletes had elevated serum troponin I levels or diagnostic ST/T wave changes on ECG and biventricular size and function were both normal on TTE and CMR.

CMR abnormalities detected in convalescent COVID-19 raised concerns for long-term CV complications even in asymptomatic patients. However, the clinical significance of these findings remains uncertain and further studies are needed to confirm the clinical role of imaging in a long-term setting. The potential role of CMR in screening athletes is debated in the literature.[69] The COVID-HEART trial is an ongoing multicentre UK trial, which will clarify the association of COVID-19–related cardiac involvement with co-morbidity, genetics, patient-reported quality of life measures, and functional capacity.[70]

Table 1 summarizes the studies of TTE and CMR findings in patients with COVID-19.

Computed Tomography

For patients with active COVID-19 and non-ST-elevation MI, noninvasive diagnostic testing before catheterization was recommended during the pandemic.[71] In hemodynamically stable cases with low or intermediate CV risk, computed tomography coronary angiography (CTCa) could be considered as an alternative to invasive coronary angiogram.[72] CTCa also provides information on lung parenchyma and pulmonary vessels, while excluding significant coronary artery disease with almost 100% negative predictive value.[73]

A retrospective study of 100 COVID-19 patients who underwent computed tomography pulmonary angiography (CTPA) showed that 23% had acute pulmonary embolism (PE).[74] Those with PE had more severe disease requiring more intensive care admissions and mechanical ventilation (PE vs non-PE: 74% vs 22%, and 65% vs 25% respectively, $P = .001$ for both comparisons). These findings were confirmed by several studies[22,40,75] highlighting the important diagnostic and prognostic role of CTPA in COVID-19 patients. Moreover, the detection of subepicardial hyperattenuation in contrast-enhanced computed tomography combined with cardiac gating can be useful in the evaluation of COVID-19 patients with suspected myocarditis.[76]

CARDIOVASCULAR EFFECTS OF DRUGS AND VACCINES AGAINST SARS-CoV-2: IS THERE A ROLE FOR CARDIAC IMAGING?

Chloroquine and hydroxychloroquine are well established treatments in non-CV conditions and have now been used in the treatment of COVID-19.[77,78] Although there are inconsistent data regarding their efficacy, and large, randomized controlled trials are needed to establish their use in clinical practice, they are widely known to cause arrhythmias.[79,80] Azithromycin used in combination with hydroxychloroquine is known to prolong QT interval.[81] A retrospective cohort study of 1438 patients hospitalized with COVID-19 showed that cardiac arrest was more likely in patients receiving both hydroxychloroquine and azithromycin than in patients receiving neither drug.[82] In the clinical scenarios of arrhythmia, CMR plays an important role in risk stratification identifying possible pathologic substrates (myocardial edema, ischemia, fibrosis) in patients with new onset arrhythmias.

Cases of thromboembolic events associated with thrombocytopenia have been reported after vaccination with both ChadOx1 nCoV-19 AZD1222 (AstraZeneca COVID-19 vaccine) and Ad26.COV2.S (Janssen COVID-19 vaccine).[28,29]

Cases of myocarditis and pericarditis have also been reported after mRNA vaccines, BNTb162 (Pfizer) and mRNA-1273 (Moderna),[30,83–85] but similar pattern of these complications have not been reported after Ad26.COV2.S (Janssen

Table 1
Studies of imaging findings (TTE/CMR) in patients with COVID-19

Authors	Study Design	Imaging Modality	Population	Results
Giustino et al,[35] 2020	International, multicenter retrospective study Cardiac Injury Research in COVID-19 Registry (CRIC-19)	TTE	N = 305 hospitalized patients with COVID-19 Age, range (y): 63 (53–73) Male/Female, n: 205/305	Myocardial injury was observed in 190 patients (62.3%) TTE abnormal in 2/3rds of patients with myocardial injury: <ul><li>LV wall motion abnormalities (N = 45, 23.7%)</li><li>LV global dysfunction (N = 35, 18.4%)</li><li>RV dysfunction (N = 50, 26.3%)</li><li>Pericardial effusion (N = 22, 7.2%)</li><li>Diastolic dysfunction grade II or III (N = 25, 13.2%)</li></ul> In-hospital mortality: <ul><li>5.2% in patients without myocardial injury</li><li>18.6% in patients with myocardial injury and without TTE abnormalities</li><li>31.7% in patients with myocardial injury and TTE abnormalities</li></ul>
Dweck et al,[36] 2020	Prospective international survey (www.escardio.org/eacvi/surveys)	TTE	N = 1216 hospitalized patients with COVID-19, 69 countries Age, range (y): 62 (52–71) Male/Female, n: 844/365	667 (55%) patients had abnormal TTE: <ul><li>39% LV abnormalities (predominantly not specific)</li><li>33% RV abnormalities (more common in patients with more severe COVID-19)</li></ul>

(continued on next page)

Table 1
(continued)

Authors	Study Design	Imaging Modality	Population	Results
				• 14% severe LV, RV, or bi-ventricular systolic dysfunction Independent predictors of LV abnormalities: elevated NPs (OR 2.96; 95% CI, 1.75–5.05) and troponin (OR 1.69; 95% CI, 1.13–2.53) Independent predictor of RV abnormalities: severity of COVID-19 symptoms (OR 3.19; 95% CI, 1.73–6.10)
Szekely et al,[37] 2020	Prospective observational single-center study	TTE	N = 100 hospitalized patients with COVID-19 Age, mean ± SD (y): 66.1 ± 17.3 Male/Female, n: 63/37	68 (68%) patients had abnormal TTE: • 39% RV dilatation ± dysfunction • 16% LV diastolic dysfunction • 10% LV systolic dysfunction • 3% valvular heart disease 60% among deteriorating patients had RV dilatation and dysfunction (+/-DVT)
Kim et al,[43] 2020	Prospective Multicenter Registry	TTE	N = 510 hospitalized patients with COVID-19 Age, mean ± SD (y): 64 ± 14 Male/Female, n: 335/175	• 35% RV dilatation • 15% RV dysfunction • RV dysfunction increased step-wise with RV dilatation • Adverse RV remodeling pre-dicted mortality independent of clinical and biomarker risk stratification (HR 2.73; 95% CI, 1.72–4.35; P < .001)
Li et al,[44] 2020	Prospective observational single-center study	TTE	N = 120 hospitalized patients with COVID-19	RVLS was a powerful predictor of higher mortality in patients

Study	Study design	Modality	Population	Findings
			Age, mean ± SD (y): 61 ± 14 Male/Female, n: 57/63 N = 37 healthy volunteers	with COVID-19 (HR 1.33; 95% CI, 1.15–1.53; $P < .001$) The best cut-off value of RVLS for prediction of outcome was −23% (AUC: 0.87; $P < .001$; sensitivity, 94.4%; specificity, 64.7%).
Goerlich et al,[53] 2020	Retrospective observational single-center study	TTE	N = 75 hospitalized patients with COVID-19 Cases (n = 39): basal LS <13.9% (absolute value) Controls (n = 36): basal LS >13.9% (absolute value) Age, mean ± SD (y): 61.9 ± 13.5 Male/Female, n: 44/31	52% had a reduced basal strain on STE (basal LS 10.0 ± 2.9% vs 16.9 ± 2.3%, $P < .001$) GLS was significantly lower in COVID-19 cases vs controls (13.9 ± 4.1% vs 18.8 ± 2.7%, $P < .001$) LVEF (%) was similar between groups (62.5 [55.0–64.4] vs 57.5 [47.5–62.5], $P = .11$
Puntmann et al,[63] 2020	Prospective observational single-center study	CMR	N = 100 patients recovered from COVID-19, CMR 71 (64–92) days from positive test Age, mean ± SD (y): 49 ± 14 Male/Female:53/47 N = 50 age and sex matched healthy controls N = 57 risk factor matched controls	Patients recovered from COVID-19 had lower LVEF and RVEF, higher LVEDVi, and raised native T1 and T2 values compared with both control groups. Greater proportions of patients with ischemic (32% vs 17%) and nonischemic (20% vs 7%) LGE patterns than the risk factor matched control group. There was a greater proportion of cases with pericardial enhancement (22% vs 14%) and pericardial effusion (20% vs 7%) compared with the risk factor matched control group.
Huang et al,[64] 2020	Retrospective observational single-center study	CMR	N = 26 patients recovered from moderate-severe COVID-19 Age, range (y): 38 (32–45) Male/Female: 10/16	58% had abnormal CMR: • Myocardial edema in 14 patients (54%) • LGE in 8 patients (31%)

(continued on next page)

Table 1
(continued)

Authors	Study Design	Imaging Modality	Population	Results
			N = 20 age and sex matched healthy controls	Global native T1, T2, and ECV values were significantly elevated in recovered COVID-19 patients with positive conventional CMR findings, compared with patients without positive findings and healthy controls Decreased RV function parameters (RVEF, RVCO, RVCI, and RVSV) were found in patients with positive conventional CMR findings, compared with healthy controls ($P < .05$)
Kotecha et al,[65] 2021	Prospective observational multicentre study	CMR	N = 148 recovered COVID-19 patients (moderate-severe COVID-19) Age mean ± SD (y): 64 ± 12 Male/Female: 104/44 N = 40 risk factor matched controls N = 40 healthy volunteers	• LV function was normal in 89% • Myocarditis-like scar noted in 26% • Infarction and/or ischemia in 22% • Dual pathology in 6% No difference in LVEDVi, LVESVi, LVEF between recovered COVID-19 patients and risk factor matched controls. No difference in native T1, T2 values between recovered COVID-19 patients and risk factor matched controls. Higher proportion of subepicardial LGE noted in recovered COVID-19 patients compared with risk factor matched controls (22% vs 5%, $P = .018$).

				Higher levels of RVEDVi, RVESVi, RVEF noted in recovered COVID-19 patients compared with risk factor matched controls
Rajpal et al,[66] 2021	Case Series (single centre)	TTE, CMR	N = 26 competitive college athletes recovered from COVID-19 (14 asymptomatic, 12 mild symptoms) Age, mean ± SD (y): 19.5 ± 1.5 Male/Female: 15/11	Normal biventricular size and function by TTE and CMR None had troponin elevation or diagnostic ST/T wave changes on ECG 4 athletes (15%) met the updated LLC for clinically suspected myocarditis 8 athletes (30%) had nonspecific LGE
Starekova et al,[67] 2021	Case Series (single centre)	TTE, CMR	N = 145 competitive college athletes recovered from COVID-19 (17% asymptomatic, 49% mild, 28% moderate symptoms) Age, range (y): 20 (17–23) Male/Female: 108/37	TTE was unremarkable 2 athletes (1.4%) had myocarditis by LLC, troponin abnormal in the more severe case 40 patients (27.6%) had small nonspecific foci of LGE
Gorecka et al,[70] 2021 COVID-HEART Investigators	Prospective observational multicentre study (COVID-HEART study)	CMR	*Inclusion criteria:* hospitalized patient population (age ≥18 y), or those recently discharged from hospital (within 28 d after discharge), with a diagnosis of COVID-19 *Exclusion criteria:* unable or unwilling to consent, contraindication to CMR, pregnancy or breast-feeding *Risk factor matched controls:* matched on age and CVD risk factors cohort	Ongoing trial

AUC, area under the receiver operating characteristic curve; CI, confidence interval; CMR, cardiac magnetic resonance; COVID-19, coronavirus disease 2019; DVT, deep vein thrombosis; ECG, electrocardiogram; ECV, extracellular volume fraction; GLS, global longitudinal strain; HR, hazard ratio; LGE, late gadolinium enhancement; LLC, Lake Louise criteria; LS, longitudinal strain; LV, left ventricular; LVEDVi, left ventricular end-diastolic volume index; LVEF, left ventricular ejection fraction; LVESVi, left ventricular end-systolic volume index; NPs, natriuretic peptides; OR, odds ratio; RV, right ventricular; RVCI, right ventricular cardiac index; RVCO, right ventricular cardiac output; RVEDVi, right ventricular end-diastolic volume index; RVEF, right ventricular ejection fraction; RVESVi, right ventricular end-systolic volume index; RVLS, right ventricular longitudinal strain; RVSV, right ventricular stroke volume; SD, standard deviation; STE, speckle tracking echocardiography; TTE, transthoracic echocardiogram.

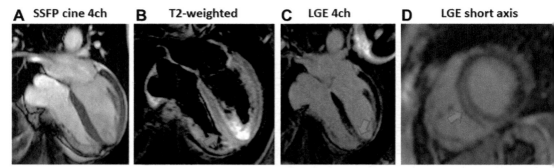

Fig. 5. CMR findings in a 46-year-old lady with acute myocarditis 1 week after the second dose of mRNA-127₇ (Moderna vaccine), who was admitted with chest pain, high troponin T levels (113 ng/L, cut off 14 ng/L), and in ferolateral T-wave inversion on electrocardiogram (ECG). Computed tomography pulmonary angiogram (CTPA) was negative for pulmonary embolism. (*A*) Steady-state free precession (SSFP) MRI cine 4 chamber (4ch) showin mild impairment of left ventricular systolic function. (*B*) T2-weighted imaging showing high signal suggestive e myocardial edema (*arrow*) in the apical septum. (*C, D*) Late gadolinium enhancement (LGE) imaging 4 chanbe (4ch) and short axis showing midwall LGE in the apical septum matching the relevant myocardial edema.

COVID-19 vaccine). However, presentations were mild, none with evidence of acute SARS-CoV-2 infection, nor met criteria for MIS. The CMR findings were consistent with myocarditis in all cases highlighting the role of CMR in detecting pathology even in less aggressive diseases. **Fig. 5** shows the CMR findings of a patient admitted with acute myocarditis 1 week after mRNA-1273 vaccination.

SUMMARY

Advanced cardiac imaging plays an essential role in the diagnosis, prognosis, and management of COVID-19 patients. It provides noninvasive tools for the recognition of the broad spectrum of CV complications in COVID-19, along with the potential CV side effects of the available vaccinations against SARS-CoV-2. However, the clinical significance of the imaging findings after COVID-19 recovery remains unclear and needs further study in large, randomized clinical trials.

CLINICS CARE POINTS

- Cardiovascular (CV) disease increases the risk of severe COVID-19 presentation.
- CV manifestations may occur during the acute phase of COVID-19, and cardiac involvement appears to be correlated with COVID-19 severity.
- Evidence suggests sustained CV involvement is uncommon. Even if patients have scar, structural and functional abnormalities, there is no difference to carefully matched control groups in the entire COVID-19 severity spectrum.

- CV involvement in athletes after COVID-19 is rare.
- There may be a link between mRNA vaccines and myocarditis, but the clinical course seems benign. More evidence is needed.

DISCLOSURES

E. Nakou, E. De Garate, K. Liang, and M. William have nothing to disclose. C. Bucciarelli-Ducci i the chief executive officer (CEO; part-time) of th Society for Cardiovascular Magnetic Resonanc (SCMR); she received speakers fees from Circ Cardiovascular Imaging. D.J. Pennell receive research support from Siemens, and speaker fees from Circle, Bayer, and Chiesi.

REFERENCES

1. World Health Organization. Coronavirus Diseas 2019 (COVID-19) Situation Report-51. 2020. Ava able at: https://www.who.int/docs/default-source coronaviruse/situation-reports/20200311-sitrep-51- covid-19.pdf. Accessed 28 January, 2021.
2. Bonow RO, Fonarow GC, O'Gara PT, et al. Associa tion of coronovirus disease 2019 (COVID-19) wi myocardial injury and mortality. JAMA Cardi 2020;5:751–3.
3. Driggin E, Madhavan MV, Bikdeli B, et al. Cardiova cular considerations for patients, health car workers, and health systems during the COVID-1 pandemic. J Am Coll Cardiol 2020;75:2352–71.
4. Li B, Yang J, Zhao F, et al. Prevalence and impact c cardiovascular metabolic disease on COVID-19 i China. Clin Res Cardiol 2020;109:531–8.
5. Zhou F, Yu T, Du R, et al. Clinical course and risk fac tor for mortality of adult inpatients with COVID-19 i

Wuhan, China: a retrospective cohort study. Lancet 2020;395:1054–62.

6. Hu H, Ma F, Wei X, et al. Coronavirus fulminant myocarditis saved with glucocorticoid and human immunoglobulin. Eur Heart J 2021;42:206. https://doi.org/10.1093/eurheartj/ehaa190.

7. Bangalore S, Sharma A, Slotwiner A, et al. ST-segment elevation in patients with covid-19- A case series. N Engl J Med 2020;382:2478–80.

8. Tsao CW, Strom JB, Chang JD, et al. COVID-19-Associated stress (Takotsubo) cardiomyopathy. Circ Cardiovasc Imaging 2020;13:e011222. https://doi.org/10.1161/CIRCIMAGING.120.011222.

9. Chen T, Wu D, Chen H, et al. Clinical characteristics of 113 deceased patients with coronavirus disease 2019: retrospective study. BMJ 2020;368. m1091.

0.. Chang WT, Toh HS, Liao CT, et al. Cardiac involvement of COVID-19: a comprehensive review. Am J Med Sci 2020;361:14–22.

1. Lax SF, Skok K, Zechner P, et al. Pulmonary arterial thrombosis in COVID-19 with fatal outcome: results from a prospective, single-center, clinicopathologic case series. Ann Intern Med 2020;173:350–61.

2. Tavazzi G, Pellegrini C, Maurelli M, et al. Myocardial localization of coronavirus in COVID-19 cardiogenic shock. Eur J Heart Fail 2020;22:911–5.

3. Lindner D, Fitzek A, Brauninger H, et al. Association of cardiac infection with SARS-CoV-2 in confirmed COVID-19 autopsy cases. JAMA Cardiol 2020;5:1281–5.

4. Puelles VG, Lütgehetmann M, Lindenmeyer MT, et al. Multiorgan and renal tropism of SARS-CoV-2. N Engl J Med 2020;383:590–2.

5. Escher F, Pietsch H, Aleshcheva G, et al. Detection of viral SARS-CoV-2 genomes and histopathological changes in endomyocardial biopsies. ESC Heart Fail 2020;7:2440–7.

6. Xu Z, Shi L, Wang Y, et al. Pathological findings of COVID-19 associated with acute respiratory distress syndrome. Lancet Respir Med 2020;8:420–2.

7. Oudit GY, Kassiri Z, Jiang C, et al. SARS-coronavirus modulation of myocardial ACE2 expression and inflammation in patients with SARS. Eur J Clin Invest 2009;39:618–25.

8. Vaduganathan M, Vardeny O, Michel T, et al. Renin-angiotensin-aldosterone system inhibitors in patients with covid-19. N Engl J Med 2020;382:1653–9.

9. Grimes JM, Grimes KV. p38 MAPK inhibition: a promising therapeutic approach for COVID-19. J Mol Cell Cardiol 2020;144:63–5.

0. Violi F, Pastori D, Pignatelli P, et al. SARS-CoV-2 and myocardial injury: a role for Nox2? Intern Emerg Med 2020;15:755–8.

1. Varga Z, Flammer AJ, Steiger P, et al. Endothelial cell infection and endotheliitis in COVID-19. Lancet 2020;395:1417–8.

22. Helms J, Tacquard C, Severac F, et al. High risk of thrombosis in patients with severe SARS-CoV-2 infection: a multicenter prospective cohort study. Intensive Care Med 2020;46:1089–98.

23. Lee CCE, Ali K, Connell D, et al. COVID-19-Associated cardiovascular complications. Diseases 2021;9:47. https://doi.org/10.3390/diseases9030047.

24. Panigada M, Bottino N, Tagliabue P, et al. Hypercoagulability of COVID-19 patients in intensive care unit: a report of thromboelastography findings and other parameters of hemostasis. J Thromb Haemost 2020;18:1738–42.

25. Lala A, Johnson K, Januzzi JL, et al. Prevalence and impact of myocardial injury in patients hospitalized with COVID-19 infection. J Am Coll Cardiol 2020;76:533–46.

26. Catapano F, Marchitelli L, Cundari G, et al. Role of advanced imaging in COVID-19 cardiovascular complications. Insights Imaging 2021;12:28. https://doi.org/10.1186/s13244-021-00973-z.

27. Nishiga M, Wang DW, Han Y, et al. COVID-19 and cardiovascular disease: from basic mechanisms to clinical perspectives. Nat Rev Cardiol 2020;17:543–58.

28. Schultz NH, Sørvoll IH, Michelsen AE, et al. Thrombosis and thrombocytopenia after ChAdOx1 nCoV-19 vaccination. N Engl J Med 2021;384:2124–30.

29. See I, Su JR, Lale A, et al. Case reports of cerebral venous sinus thrombosis with thrombocytopenia after Ad26.COV2.S vaccination, March 2 to April 21, 2021. JAMA 2021;325:2448–56.

30. EMA. Meeting highlights from the Pharmacovigilance Risk Assessment Committee (PRAC) 3-6 May 2021 Internet Document : 7 May 2021. https://www.ema.europa.eu/en/news/meeting-highlights-pharmacovigilance-risk-assessment-committee-prac-3-6-may-2021.

31. Greinacher A, Thiele T, Warkentin TE, et al. Thrombotic thrombocytopenia after ChAdOx1 nCov-19 vaccination. N Engl J Med 2021;384:2092–101.

32. EMA. Meeting highlights from the Pharmacovigilance Risk Assessment Committee (PRAC) 3-6 May 2021 Internet Document : 7 May 2021. Available at: https://www.ema.europa.eu/en/news/meeting-highlights-pharmacovigilance-risk-assessment-committee-prac-3-6-may-2021.

33. Wang D, Hu B, Hu C, et al. Clinical characteristics of 138 hospitalized patients with 2019 novel coronavirus-infected pneumonia in Wuhan, China. JAMA 2020;323:1601–69.

34. Deng O, Hu B, Zhang Y, et al. Suspected myocardial injury in patients with COVID-19: evidence from front-line clinical observation in Wuhan, China. Int J Cardiol 2020;311:116–21.

35. Giustino G, Croft LB, Stefanini GG, et al. Characterization of myocardial injury in patients with COVID-19. J Am Coll Cardiol 2020;76:2043–55.

36. Dweck MR, Bularga A, Hahn RT, et al. Global evaluation of echocardiography in patients with COVID-19. Eur Heart J Cardiovasc Imaging 2020;21: 949–58.

37. Szekely Y, Lichter Y, Taieb P, et al. Spectrum of cardiac manifestations in COVID-19: a systematic echocardiographic study. Circulation 2020;142:342–53.

38. Fayssoil A, Mustafic H, Mansencal N. The right ventricle in COVID-19 patients. Am J Cardiol 2020; 130:166–7.

39. Creel-Bulos C, Hockstein M, Amin N, et al. Acute cor pulmonale in critically ill patients with Covid-19. N Engl J Med 2020;382:e70. https://doi.org/10. 1056/NEJMc2010459.

40. Poissy J, Goutay J, Caplan M, et al. Pulmonary embolism in patients with COVID-19: Awareness of an increased prevalence. Circulation 2020;142:184–6.

41. Ullah W, Saeed R, Sarwar U, et al. COVID-19 complicated by acute pulmonary embolism and right-Sided heart failure. JACC Case Rep 2020;2: 1379–82.

42. Himebauch AS, Yehya N, Wang Y, et al. New or persistent right ventricular systolic dysfunction is associated with worse outcomes in pediatric acute respiratory distress syndrome. Pediatr Crit Care Med 2020;21:e121–8.

43. Kim J, Volodarskiy A, Sultana R, et al. Prognostic utility of right ventricular remodelling over conventional risk stratification in patients with COVID-19. J Am Coll Cardiol 2020;76:1965–77.

44. Li Y, Li H, Zhu S, et al. Prognostic value of right ventricular longitudinal strain in patients with COVID-19. JACC Cardiovasc Imaging 2020;13:2287–99.

45. Sauer F, Dagrenat C, Couppie P, et al. Pericardial effusion in patients with COVID-19: case series. Eur Hear J Case Rep 2020;4(FI1):1–7.

46. Blagojevic NR, Bosnjakovic D, Vukomanovic V, et al. Acute pericarditis and SARS-CoV-2: case report. Int J Infect Dis 2020;101:180–2.

47. Purohit R, Kanwal A, Pandit A, et al. Acute myopericarditis with pericardial effusion and cardiac tamponade in a patient with COVID-19. Am J Case Rep 2020;21:e925554. https://doi.org/10.12659/AJCR. 925554.

48. Dabbagh MF, Aurora L, D'Souza P, et al. Cardiac tamponade secondary to COVID-19. JACC Case Rep 2020;2:1326–30.

49. Hua A, O'Gallagher K, Sado D, et al. Life-threatening cardiac tamponade complicating myo-pericarditis in COVID-19. Eur Heart J 2020;41:2130. https://doi. org/10.1093/eurheartj/ehaa253.

50. Pastore MC, De Carli G, Mandoli GE, et al. The prognostic role of speckle tracking echocardiography in clinical practice: evidence and reference values from the literature. Heart Fail Rev 2020. https://doi. org/10.1007/s10741-020-09945-9. Online ahead of print.

51. Jahn L, Kramann R, Marx N, et al. Speckle tracking echocardiography and all-cause and cardiovascular mortality risk in Chronic kidney disease patients. Kidney Blood Press Res 2019;44:690–703.

52. Janus SE, Hajjari J, Karnib M, et al. Prognostic value of left ventricular global longitudinal strain in COVID-19. Am J Cardiol 2020;131:134–6.

53. Goerlich E, Gilotra NA, Minhas AS, et al. Prominent longitudinal strain reduction of basal left ventricular segments in patients with coronavirus disease-19. J Card Fail 2020;27:100–4.

54. Allen BD, Wong TC, Bucciarelli-Ducci C, et al. Society for Cardiovascular Magnetic Resonance (SCMR) guidance for re-activation of cardiovascular magnetic resonance practice after peak phase of the COVID-19 pandemic. J Cardiovasc Magn Reson 2020;22:58. https://doi.org/10.1186/s12968-020-00654-8.

55. Petersen S, Friedrich MG, Leiner T, et al. Cardiovascular magnetic resonance for patients with coronavirus disease 2019 (COVID-19). JACC CVI 2021 in press.

56. Kelle S, Bucciarelli-Ducci C, Judd RM, et al. Society for Cardiovascular Magnetic Resonance (SCMR) recommended CMR protocols for scanning patients with active or convalescent phase COVID-19 infection. J Cardiovasc Magn Reson 2020;22:61. https: doi.org/10.1186/s12968-020-00656-6.

57. Mahrholdt H, Wagner A, Judd RM, et al. Delayed enhancement cardiovascular magnetic resonance assessment of non-ischaemic cardiomyopathies. Eur Heart 2005;26:1461–74.

58. Friedrich MG, Sechtem U, Schulz-Menger J, et al. Cardiovascular magnetic resonance in myocarditis: a JACC white paper. JACC 2009;53:1475–87.

59. Ferreira VM, Schulz-Menger J, Holmvang G, et al. Cardiovascular magnetic resonance in nonischemic myocardial inflammation: expert recommendations. J Am Coll Cardiol 2018;72:3158–76.

60. Demirkiran A, Everaars H, Amier RP, et al. Cardiovascular magnetic resonance techniques for tissue characterization after acute myocardial injury. Eur Heart J Cardiovasc Imaging 2020;20:723–34.

61. Ghadri JR, Wittstein IS, Prasad A, et al. International expert consensus document on takotsubo syndrome (part i): clinical characteristics, diagnostic criteria, and pathophysiology. Eur Heart J 2018;39: 2032–46.

62. Jabri A, Kalra A, Kumar A, et al. Incidence of stress cardiomyopathy during the coronavirus disease 2019 pandemic. JAMA Netw Open 2020;3: e2014780.

63. Puntmann VO, Carerj ML, Wieters I, et al. Outcomes of cardiovascular magnetic resonance imaging in patients recently recovered from coronavirus disease 2019 (COVID-19). JAMA Cardiol 2020;5: 1265–73.

4. Huang L, Zhao P, Tang D, et al. Cardiac involvement in patients recovered from COVID-2019 identified using magnetic resonance imaging. JACC Cardiovasc Imaging 2020;13:2330–9.

5. Kotecha T, Knight DS, Razvi Y, et al. Patterns of myocardial injury in recovered troponin-positive COVID-19 patients assessed by cardiovascular magnetic resonance. Eur Heart J 2021;42:1866–78.

6. Rajpal S, Tong MS, Borchers J, et al. Cardiovascular magnetic resonance findings in competitive athletes recovering from COVID-19 infection. JAMA Cardiol 2021;6:116–8.

7. Starekova J, Bluemke DA, Bradham WS, et al. Evaluation for myocarditis in competitive student athletes recovering from coronavirus disease 2019 with cardiac magnetic resonance imaging. JAMA Cardiol 2021;6:945–50.

8. Martinez MW, Tucker AM, Bloom OJ, et al. Prevalence of inflammatory heart disease among professional athletes with prior COVID-19 infection who received systematic return-to-play cardiac screening. JAMA Cardiol 2021;6:745–52.

9. Phelan D, Kim JH, Elliott MD, et al. Screening of potential cardiac involvement in competitive athletes recovering from COVID-19: an expert consensus statement. JACC Cardiovasc Imaging 2020;13: 2635–52.

10. Gorecka M, McCann GP, Berry C, et al. Demographic, multi-morbidity and genetic impact on myocardial involvement and its recovery from COVID-19: protocol design of COVID-HEART-a UK, multicentre, observational study. J Cardiovasc Magn Reson 2021;23:77. https://doi.org/10.1186/s12968-021-00752-1.

11. Long B, Brady WJ, Koyfman A, et al. Cardiovascular complications in COVID-19. Am J Emerg Med 2020; 38:1504–7.

12. Pontone G, Baggiano A, Conte E, et al. "Quadruple rule out" with cardiac computed tomography in COVID-19 patient with equivocal acute coronary syndrome presentation. JACC Cardiovasc Imaging 2020;13:1854–6.

13. Agricola E, Beneduce A, Esposito A, et al. Heart and lung multimodality imaging in COVID-19. JACC Cardiovasc Imaging 2020;13:1792–808.

14. Grillet F, Behr J, Calame P, et al. Acute pulmonary embolism associated with COVID-19 pneumonia detected by pulmonary CT angiography. Radiology 2020;296:E186–8.

75. Leonard-Lorant I, Delabranche X, Severac F, et al. Acute pulmonary embolism in COVID-19 patients on CT angiography and relationship to D-dimer levels. Radiology 2020;296:E189–91.

76. Singh V, Choi AD, Leipsic J, et al. Use of cardiac CT amidst the COVID-19 pandemic and beyond: North American perspective. J Cardiovasc Comput Tomogr 2020;15:16–26.

77. Gautret P, Lagier JC, Parola P, et al. Hydroxychloroquine and azithromycin as a treatment of COVID-19: results of an open-label non-randomized clinical trial. Int J Antimicrob Agents 2020;56:105949.

78. Wang M, Cao R, Zhang L, et al. Remdesivir and chloroquine effectively inhibit the recently emerged novel coronavirus (2019-nCoV) in vitro. Cell Res 2020;30:269–71.

79. Roden DM, Harrington RA, Poppas A, et al. Considerations for drug interactions on QTc in exploratory COVID-19 treatment. Circulation 2020;141:e906–7.

80. Mercuro NJ, Yen CF, Shim DJ, et al. Risk of QT interval prolongation associated with use of hydroxychloroquine with or without concomitant azithromycin among hospitalized patients testing positive for coronavirus disease 2019 (COVID-19). JAMA Cardiol 2020;5:1036–41.

81. Hancox JC, Hasnain M, Vieweg WV, et al. Azithromycin, cardiovascular risks, QTc interval prolongation, Torsade de Pointes, and regulatory issues: a narrative review based on the study of case reports. Ther Adv Infect Dis 2013;1:155–65.

82. Rosenberg ES, Dufort EM, Udo T, et al. Association of treatment with hydroxychloroquine or azithromycin with in- hospital mortality in patients with COVID-19 in New York state. JAMA 2020;323: 2493–502.

83. Gargano JW, Wallace M, Hadler SC, et al. Use of mRNA COVID-19 vaccine after reports of myocarditis among vaccine recipients: update from the advisory committee on immunization practices - United States, June 2021. MMWR Morb Mortal Wkly Rep 2021;70:977–82.

84. Dickey JB, Albert E, Badr M, et al. A series of patients with myocarditis following SARS-CoV-2 vaccination with mRNA-1279 and BNT162b2. JACC Cardiovasc Imaging 2021;14:1862–3.

85. Shaw KE, Cavalcante JL, Han BK, et al. Possible association between COVID-19 vaccine and myocarditis: clinical and CMR findings. JACC Cardiovasc Imaging 2021;14:1856–61.

Arrhythmogenic Risk and Mechanisms of QT-Prolonging Drugs to Treat COVID-19

Marco Schiavone, MD[a],*, Alessio Gasperetti, MD[a,b], Elisa Gherbesi, MD[a], Luca Bergamaschi, MD[a], Roberto Arosio, MD[a], Gianfranco Mitacchione, MD, PhD[a], Maurizio Viecca, MD[a], Giovanni B. Forleo, MD, PhD[a]

KEYWORDS

- QT interval • COVID-19 • Ventricular arrhythmias • Torsade de point • Hydroxychloroquine
- Antivirals

KEY POINTS

- COVID-19 patients might experience an increased arrhythmic risk due to QT prolongation, as for their clinical status or for the massive off-label use of potentially QT-prolonging drugs.
- In such patients, a complete baseline QT assessment at a 12-lead ECG should be performed, as well as with Tisdale score calculation and ECG monitoring during drug administration.
- Among the most important clinical factors predisposing to QT prolongation and ventricular arrhythmias, genetic predisposition, older age, female gender, electrolyte disorders, pharmacologic interactions, and bradycardia represent the most relevant features.
- Chloroquine and hydroxychloroquine are associated with QT prolongation especially when used in combination with macrolides, such as azithromycin, or fluoroquinolones.
- A scarce body of evidence exists on antivirals and immunomodulators, with lopinavir/ritonavir appearing to be the most frequently associated with QT prolongation.

INTRODUCTION

Apart from a well-known respiratory involvement,[1,2] several reports have described the presence of a significant myocardial injury in coronavirus disease (COVID-19), often sustained by macrothrombosis and microthrombosis, as well as a direct cardiac damage.[3–10] Indeed, as highlighted in different studies, acute coronary syndromes and cardiac arrhythmias have been reported as potential complications in hospitalized patients, often impairing COVID-19 patients' prognosis.[11–18] Besides a disease-related cardiac involvement, the massive off-label use of several drugs,[19,20] including immunosuppressive agents (eg, anakinra or tocilizumab), different antivirals (eg, oseltamivir, remdesivir, or the lopinavir/ritonavir combination), and antimalarial drugs such as chloroquine (CQ) and hydroxychloroquine (HCQ) with or without azithromycin (AM), has generated concerns in the early phase of the pandemic because of their possible arrhythmogenic effects in relation to QT interval prolongation. Indeed, some of these drugs have never been used on a large scale and little is known about their possible arrhythmogenic effects in elderly, critically ill patients, often showing multiple comorbidities, being treated with multiple drugs. Most of these drugs

[a] Cardiology Unit, Luigi Sacco University Hospital, Milan, Italy; [b] Division of Cardiology, Johns Hopkins University, Baltimore, MD, USA
* Corresponding author: Luigi Sacco University Hospital, Via G.B. Grassi 74, Milan 20157, Italy.
E-mail address: marco.schiavone11@gmail.com

Card Electrophysiol Clin 14 (2022) 95–104
https://doi.org/10.1016/j.ccep.2021.10.009
1877-9182/22/© 2021 Elsevier Inc. All rights reserved.

may prolong the QT interval both with direct (channel blocking activity) or indirect effects (eg, liver and/or kidney toxicity, cytochrome interactions, electrolyte imbalance), potentially increasing the arrhythmic (eg, *Torsade de Pointes* [TdP]) and nonarrhythmic mortality. The aim of this work is to summarize the underlying arrhythmogenic mechanisms related to the use of potentially QT-prolonging drugs used during the COVID-19 pandemic.

THE QT INTERVAL

The QT interval is the interval from the beginning of ventricular depolarization to the completion of the repolarization of the entire ventricular mass. Ideally, the QT interval should be measured at a paper rate of 25 mm/s from the beginning of the QRS until the return to baseline of the T wave. The QT interval should be calculated in a total of 6 leads, with 3 leads taken from peripheral leads (avoiding DIII and aVR because of frequent low voltages and inverted polarity, respectively) and 3 precordial leads (preferably V2, V4, and V6). The QT value should be derived from the median of the 6 individual leads. Although QT calculation is a well-known and standardized methodology, a correct and consistent measurement of the QT interval is always difficult to obtain in clinical practice. Deciding if QT interval is normal or prolonged is often challenging, as reported by Viskin and colleagues, underlining that most physicians, including many cardiologists, cannot accurately calculate a QT and cannot correctly identify a long QT.[21] Moreover, as the heart rate is the major determinant of the QT interval, a corrected QT interval value (QTc) should always be preferred in clinical practice. Several formulae may commonly be adopted to calculate QTc, with the Bazett formula being the most frequently used. Nevertheless, Vandenberk and colleagues[22] showed that the Bazett formula may overestimate the number of patients at potential risk of dangerous QTc prolongation when compared with Fridericia and Framingham formulae. To sum up different clinical data, the Framingham formula still seems to be the best choice to predict drug-induced QTc prolongation.[23] Different cut-offs have been traditionally proposed to define when a QTc is prolonged, with the most significantly reliable being 450 msec, with values of greater than 500 msec being considered definitely abnormal and potentially arrhythmogenic[24,25]; thus, drug-induced changes in QTc of greater than 50 msec are often used as safety endpoints when evaluating drug effects and may justify a treatment interruption. A proposed algorithm to identify patients at risk of

developing ventricular arrhythmias (VAs) whe treating with one or more QT-prolonging drug during the COVID-19 pandemic is reported **Fig. 1**.

MECHANISMS OF QT PROLONGATION

QT prolongation is associated with an increase both arrhythmic and nonarrhythmic mortality, an it is often used as a metric of drug safety.[26] Indee QT prolongation is related to a mix of modifiab and unmodifiable risk factors that may determir why at same drugs dosages, drug-induced lon QT may happen only in some cases. Dru induced effects are one of the most frequent rea sons for QT prolongation: an updated list of th medications associated with QT prolongatio and risk of TdP is reported on https://www crediblemeds.org. It should be noted that, beside the direct impact of some medications on the Q interval, drug-to-drug and drug-to-cytochrome ir teractions should always be considered, espe cially in COVID-19, when assessing the risk QT prolongation in the COVID-19 clinical setting

Nonmodifiable Risk Factors

Genetic background, as well as older age and f male gender, are the most important unmodifiab risk factors. Long QT syndrome (LQTS) represen a heterogeneous family of inherited primal arrhythmia syndromes characterized by QT inte val prolongation and T-wave abnormalities on th ECG. Patients affected by LQTS have been ident fied all over the world and in all ethnic group among Caucasians, the prevalence of LQTS h been 1:2000 apparently healthy newborns.[27] Risl of VAs related to LQTS are mainly due to adrer ergic activation, and the annual rate of sudden ca diac death (SCD) in patients with untreated LQT is estimated to be between 0.33% an 0.9%.[28,29] Mutations in 13 genes have been trad tionally associated with LQTS—among those, mu tations in potassium-channel genes KCNQ1 (LQT locus) and KCNH2 (LQT2 locus) and the sodiun channel gene SCN5A (LQT3 locus) are the mo common causes of the LQTS and account f approximately 75% of cases.[30] Once diagnos is made, risk stratification is mandatory to taile lifestyle changes and to deliver the adequate the apy, such as implantable cardioverter-defibrillate (ICD) in high-risk patients, with the modern subcu taneous ICD potentially being the most appr priate therapeutic option.[31–35] All LQTS patient regardless of the SCD risk, should avoid QT prolonging drugs, promptly correct electrolyte ab normalities (hypokalemia, hypomagnesemia, an hypocalcemia) that may occur during diarrhe

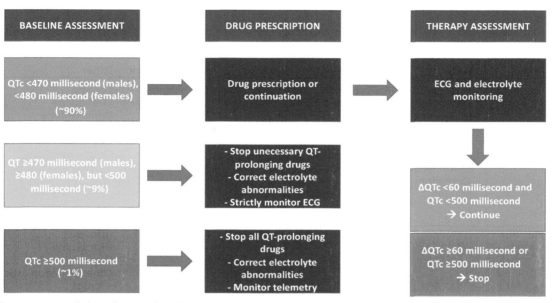

Fig. 1. Proposed algorithm to identify patients at risk of developing ventricular arrhythmias when treating with one or more QT-prolonging drugs. (*Adapted from* Giudicessi JR, Noseworthy PA, Friedman PA, Ackerman MJ. Urgent Guidance for Navigating and Circumventing the QTc-Prolonging and Torsadogenic Potential of Possible Pharmacotherapies for Coronavirus Disease 19 (COVID-19). Mayo Clin Proc. 2020;95(6):1213-1221. https://doi.org/10.1016/j.mayocp.2020.03.024; with permission)

vomiting, or metabolic conditions and avoid genotype-specific triggers for arrhythmias (strenuous swimming, especially in LQTS1, and exposure to loud noises in LQTS2 patients).[36] There are more than 260 medicines on the "drugs to avoid" list for patients with LQTS, that are generally grouped as follows:

- Known risk: drugs that should never or very rarely use because of clear danger—if administered, LQTS patients should be treated by cardiologists with expertise in arrhythmias management.
- Possible risk: drugs that have been found to increase QT interval and may be dangerous in some LQTS patients—if necessary, those drugs may be prescribed by specialists.
- Conditional risk: drugs that may increase risk in LQTS patients only in certain conditions (eg, overdose, prolonged treatments, use in combination with other drugs that may change their clearance)—most of those drugs can be prescribed safely.
- Special risk: drugs that have a theoretic risk of causing arrhythmias in LQTS patients because of their adrenergic effect—most of those drugs can be prescribed to carefully selected LQTS patients[37].

Given the pandemic nature of COVID-19, even a rare congenital genetic predisposition, may result

in tremendous consequences if undetected, in terms of drug-induced TdP and SCD. The most widely used QT-prolonging drugs that should be avoided in patients with LQTS and their associated risk have been summarized in **Table 1**.

Modifiable Risk Factors

Electrolyte abnormalities are the most common modifiable risk factors associated with QT prolongation. Among those, hypokalemia has a particular arrhythmogenic effect, not only prolonging the QT interval but also being a major risk factor for drug-induced LQTS as it increases the tendency of $K_v11.1$ channels to remain inactivated and decreases repolarizing currents. Hypocalcemia and hypomagnesemia as well may show a QT-prolonging effect. Kidney and liver failure have both been associated with the risk of QT prolongation because of their role in metabolite/toxin clearance; finally, bradycardia is a relevant additional risk factor.

Patients accessing intensive care such as COVID-19 severe infections should therefore be strictly monitored because of their potential exposure to these risk factors. Lastly, to estimate the risk of drug-induced QT prolongation, all the patients treated with a potential QT-prolonging drug should be evaluated with a Tisdale score at baseline (**Table 2**).[38] Indeed, the Tisdale risk classes are, respectively, associated with 15%, 37%,

Table 1
Most widely used potentially QT-prolonging drugs that should be avoided in patients with long QT and their associated risk.[66]

Risk	AAD	AB/AFA/AM	AP/AD	Anesthetic	Other
Known	Amiodarone Dronedarone Disopyramide Dofetilide Flecainide Ibutilide Procainamide Quinidine Sotalol	Azithromycin Ciprofloxacin Clarithromycin Erythromycin Fluconazole Gatifloxacin Levofloxacin Moxifloxacin Roxithromycin Chloroquine Hydroxychloroquine	Chlorpromazine Citalopram	Propofol Sevoflurane	Cocaine Methadone Domperidone Levosulpiride Ondansetron Other antineoplastic drugs
Possible		Norfloxacin Ofloxacin	Lithium Venlafaxine Aripiprazole Clozapine	Tramadol	Alfuzosin Nicardipine Oxytocin Other antineoplastic drugs
Conditional	Ivabradine Propafenone Ranolazine	Piperacillin/ tazobactam Amphotericin B Ketoconazole Metronidazole Voriconazole	Amisulpride Amitriptyline Fluoxetine Olanzapine Paroxetine Quetiapine Risperidone Sertraline Trazodone		Hydrochlorothiazide Torasemide Amantadine Indapamide Furosemide Loperamide Metolazone Metoclopramide Omeprazole Lansoprazole Pantoprazole Esomeprazole
Special	Drugs used for the treatment of asthma, −ADHD, or nasal congestion				

Abbreviations: AAD, antiarrhythmic drugs; AB, antibiotics; AD, antidepressants; ADHD, attention-deficit hyperactivity disorder; AFA, antifungal agents; AM, antimalarials; AP, antipsychotics.

and 73% risk of QT prolongation, and can be extremely useful for a quick but reliable baseline risk assessment.

QT-PROLONGING DRUGS AND ARRHYTHMOGENIC RISK IN COVID-19

While waiting for the massive vaccination campaign to be completed to reach the herd immunity, several drugs proposed as potential treatments are still used worldwide to treat COVID-19. However, most of these drugs are not specific and targeted against SARS-CoV-2, so that using pre-existing drugs has represented a fast and very useful strategy with known safety, characteristics, and dosage used during the early and even late phase of the pandemic.[19] If some of these drugs have been investigated for their efficacy and safety in treating COVID-19, some others are still undergoing clinical trials to test their profile. One of the main concerns regarding the use of some of these

repurposed drugs is the potential impact on the QT interval and their arrhythmogenic effects, which is particularly noteworthy because of the common coprescription of several drugs that may show combined effects on the QT interval, as well as several clinical characteristics that may eventually lead to arrhythmic manifestations.[39] The knowledge on these potential adverse events is mostly derived from the historical data collected according to the European Union Drug Regulatory Authorities (EUDRA) vigilance by the European Medical Agency (EMA). If data on chloroquine (CQ) and hydroxychloroquine (HCQ) are more robust, data on other less commonly used drugs are weaker.

Antimalarial Agents

CQ and HCQ are antimalarial drugs that inhibit lysosomes functions increasing pH and thereby blocking endosome-mediated entry. These drugs can also interfere with cell replication, viral protein

Table 2
Tisdale score to identify hospitalized patients at risk for QT interval prolongation could lead to interventions to reduce the risk of TdP[38]

Age $\geq$ 68 y Female Sex Loop Diuretic Treatment	1 point
Serum K$^+$ $\leq$ 3.5mEq/L Acute myocardial infarction Admission QTc $\geq$ 450 msec	2 points
1-QTc-prolonging drugs 2+ QTc-prolong drugs Sepsis Heart failure hospitalization	3 points

TISDALE SCORE:
Low risk ($\leq$6 points).
Intermediate risk (7–10 points).
High risk ($\geq$11 points).

glycosylation, virus assembly, and release. CQ use is restricted because of potential overdose, acute poisoning, and death, whereas HCQ (a derivative of CQ) has been demonstrated to be far less toxic than CQ.[19] In the early phase of the pandemic, these antimalarial drugs have been suggested to be effective in treating COVID-19,[40] and they have been thereby extensively used both in mild and in severe COVID-19. Randomized trials and metanalysis have, however, shown that HCQ was not effective as it was initially supposed. In the randomized, controlled, open-label RECOV-ERY trial,[41] comparing a range of possible treatments with usual care in patients hospitalized with COVID-19, patients receiving HCQ did not have a lower incidence of death at 28 days than those who received usual care. Also, the TOGETHER trial[42] showed that an early treatment with HCQ did not have any significant benefit in decreasing COVID-19–associated hospitalization or other secondary clinical outcomes. These results were confirmed by Ghazy and colleagues[43] in a metanalysis, showing that neither CQ nor HCQ were able to decrease mortality, improve virological cure, reduce the risk for noninvasive ventilation and shorten the conversion to negative polymerase chain reaction, prevent radiological progression, and affect clinical worsening of the disease. Considering this evidence, showing a complete lack of efficacy and an increase in adverse events, most American and European medical associations and drugs associations do not recommend the use of HCQ in hospitalized COVID-19 patients and in the early stages of the disease.

Nevertheless, several trials have been performed to test the cardiac safety of CQ/HCQ in the early phase of the pandemic, and although their results may now appear outdated in the light of this recent discovery of CQ/HCQ inefficacy in COVID-19, all these analyses gave the scientific community the possibility to test these drugs during a mass-use on critically ill patients. The importance of these reports is undoubtedly related to the idea that CQ and HCQ are known to be associated with a risk of QT prolongation, so that they are classified as drugs associated with TdP on the Credible Meds Web site. Hence, between 0.5% and 2% of all the side effects of these drugs reported to the European Medicines Agency (EMA) are major arrhythmic events with non-negligible rates of cardiac arrest. Moreover, is noteworthy to underline that HCQ, besides malaria, is currently used to treat discoid or systemic lupus erythematosus, rheumatoid arthritis (RA), and systemic sclerosis.

Indeed, research on this topic is beneficial to better understand its arrhythmic safety also for these patients. Specifically, Gasperetti and colleagues extensively evaluated the arrhythmic safety of HCQ in different clinical settings.[44] In this study, enrolled patients were followed in 3 different clinical settings, defined as home management, medical ward, or intensive care unit (ICU) management, depending on the COVID-19 severity, and were all tested through serial ECG monitoring. The authors concluded that HCQ administration, alone or in combination with other potentially QTc-prolonging drugs, although potentially causing only modest QTc prolongation, did not result in significant arrhythmic events, representing a safe option for patients with COVID-19 infection. Indeed, no TdP were noticed in the entire cohort, and the described ventricular fibrillation (VF) events occurred in the ICU cohort, with acute myocardial infarction as the underlying cause. These results were confirmed by 3 different studies, enrolling patients with COVID-19 treated with HCQ. First, Mazzanti and colleagues[45] did not document any life-threatening arrhythmic event, with only a modest effect on QTc prolongation, that was attributed to the short duration of HCQ treatment in COVID-19, as HCQ reaches the steady state after 180 days of HCQ therapy.[46] Therefore, caution should be adopted when extending these safety results to patients treated for several years for other indications, that could experience a more severe QTc prolongation and related arrhythmic effects. The authors recommend to always perform a baseline ECG before starting HCQ, followed by a subsequent recording "on therapy" for patients with a normal baseline QTc, with an advisable daily monitoring for patients with baseline QTc greater than 480 msec.

Furthermore, Bernardini and colleagues[47] and Chorin and colleagues[48] evaluated the safety of the HCQ plus AM combination regimen that might surely have higher proarrhythmic effects than HCQ alone. In both cohorts, a significant increase of QT interval was noted, especially in the elderly, with 8% and 23% patients treated with HCQ + AM showing a QTc greater than 500 msec, respectively. Besides this difference, if in the first cohort no arrhythmic fatalities occurred, in the second one QT prolongation has led to 1 life-threatening arrhythmia (0.4%) in the form of TdP. These dissimilarities might be due to concurrent modifiable risk factors, such as electrolyte imbalance, comorbidities, or COVID-19 severity, that could have contributed to QT prolongation. Indeed, the safety of HCQ large-scale use in acutely ill patients with multiple comorbidities, possibly receiving several QT-prolonging drugs and potentially at risk of electrolyte disbalance, still needs to be properly tested. Even if data point toward a general arrhythmic safety of HCQ, especially when used alone or in the short-term period, a baseline ECG and a periodic QTc interval monitoring should be advisable when this drug regimen is given.

Antiviral Drugs

Lopinavir/ritonavir

Lopinavir and ritonavir (LPV/RTN) are antiretroviral protease inhibitors that are used in combination to treat human immunodeficiency virus. RTN increases the half-life of LPV by inhibiting the half-life of cytochrome P450 half-life, and thereby acting as a pharmacokinetic enhancer; LPV acts against viral 3-chymotrypsin-like protease (3CLpro). This combination has shown promising in vitro results against SARS-CoV and MERS-CoV, but clinical randomized trials did show no benefit with LPV/RTN combination beyond standard of care in hospitalized adult patients with severe COVID-19.[49] Nevertheless, some researchers, interpreting the findings of this clinical trial, suggested the earlier usage of LPV/RTN in the course of the disease may be overall beneficial in some cases.[50] Therefore, the evaluation of the arrhythmogenic effects is of pivotal importance. Indeed, this combination has an intrinsic risk of ventricular tachycardia (0.03%), VF (0.03%), and TdP (0.09%) reported in the literature, according to the EUDRA vigilance from EMA. During the pandemic, Haghjoo and colleagues[51] investigated the potential QT-prolonging role of LPV/RTN, showing a significant increase in QTc during drug therapy (along with CQ, HCQ, atazanavir/ritonavir, oseltamivir, favipiravir, and remdesivir alone in combination with

AM). Nevertheless, in this cohort, TdP occurre overall rarely (n = 9; 0.385), with 4 patients treate with HCQ + AM, whereas 5 patients were treate with LPN/RTV + AM. Interestingly, in this analysi although critical QT prolongation was associate with a higher risk of TdP, only treatment wit LPN/RTV, simultaneous administration of amic darone (known to prolong QT interval[52]) or furose mide and hypokalemia could predict th occurrence of TdP in this cohort; instead, HC use was only modestly associated with Td (0.3% of patients). Other cases of QT prolongatic with LPN/RTV treatment have been described du ing the pandemic,[53] so that careful QTc duratic evaluation and monitoring should be performe at baseline and during this drug therapy to identi patients at high risk of arrhythmias.

Remdesivir

Remdesivir is an adenosine analog that inserts i self into viral RNA chains, blocking viral replicatio Although nothing has been reported in the FD and EMA databases regarding links with QT pro longation, some case reports and scarce dat have suggested that also this drug may prolon QT, as well as induce sinus bradycardia, as r ported by Gupta and colleagues.[54] It should b noted that in this case, patients were also on A while receiving remdesivir, which is well-know to prolong the QT interval. Remdesivir monothe apy has indeed shown to prolong QTc in the Hagh joo and colleagues[51] analysis, although keeping low-risk profile in terms of QT prolongation an TdP induction. Moreover, no major cardia arrhythmia events were described in the large trial assessing remdesivir efficacy and safety pro file. Nevertheless, cardiac safety of remdesivir re mains largely uncertain and these effects wer described as reversible upon stopping remdesiv therapy, caution should be taken with this antivir agent.

Favipiravir

Favipiravir is a guanine analog that selectively in hibits viral RNA-dependent RNA polymerase an it was approved for influenza and Ebola virus infec tion. Çap and colleagues[55] specifically evaluate any change in the QTc interval in patients wh were hospitalized due to COVID-19, receiving fav piravir treatment. No significant QTc prolongatic was noted with monotherapy, when compared t HCQ or HCQ + favipiravir. On the other sid Haghjoo and colleagues[51] observed a mild QT prolongation in most cases, without TdP event even if they concluded that favipiravir monothe apy was safer than other COVID-19 mediatior in terms of QTc prolongation.

Oseltamivir

Oseltamivir is an antiviral drug that inhibits neuraminidase, expressed on the viral surface, which plays an essential role in viral entry to host cells, viral release from infected cells, and subsequent viral spread. Although its role in COVID-19 is very limited, it is noteworthy to mention that Haghjoo and colleagues[51] reported that this drug may significantly prolong QTc when used in combination with HCQ, as also suggested by Çelik and colleagues.[56] No TdP were noted in these patients, as in previous preclinical models that tested oseltamivir therapy alone, as this drug is capable to inhibit both inward and outward currents.[57] However, caution should be taken when prescribing oseltamivir plus other COVID-19 medications potentially prolonging QTc during the influenza season.

Antibacterial Drugs

Azithromycin

AM, a macrolide antibacterial agent, has an established role against a broad spectrum of gram-positive and gram-negative agents, as well as act as an immunomodulator. During the COVID-19 pandemic, it has been used in combination with HCQ because of promising in vitro findings, even further clinical trials have demonstrated that the routine use of AM for reducing time to recovery or risk of hospitalization for people with suspected COVID-19 in the community was not justified.[58] AM is a well-known QT-prolonging drug, that should be avoided in all LQTS cases, even when used as a stand-alone therapy. The arrhythmogenic potential of AM has been discussed in the previous sections when assessing the combination of this drug with HCQ. Indeed, in the PRINCIPLE trial,[58] no difference was found regarding a prolonged QTc interval between the AM group and the standard care group, but a QTc interval prolongation was most common in the HCQ + AM group.

Immunomodulators

Tocilizumab

Tocilizumab (TCZ) is an anti–interleukin (IL)-6 receptor antibody that potently inhibits inflammatory activation and is used to treat RA, systemic juvenile idiopathic arthritis, and chimeric antigen receptor–cell–induced cytokine release syndrome. In a clinical trial conducted on patients with RA, Lazzerini and colleagues[59] showed that TCZ treatment was associated with a rapid and significant reduction to mean values less than 440 msec in patients who had prolonged QTc interval at baseline. This effect seems to be driven by TCZ action

against systemic inflammation, thus providing further evidence of the close correlation between the degree of systemic inflammation and QTc duration in RA patients.[60] In this light, the administration of anti–IL-6 targeted therapies (TCZ, sarilumab) to patients with COVID-19, particularly those severely ill, has been supposed not only to promote the recovery from multiorgan dysfunction but also mitigate the associated high arrhythmic risk, in the early phase of the pandemic. However, randomized trials have shown that the use of TCZ did not result in significantly better clinical status or lower mortality than placebo at 28 days, being not effective for preventing intubation or death in moderately ill hospitalized patients with COVID-19.[61,62] Specific data on the supposed antiarrhythmic effects, associated with the anti-inflammatory effects, were not specifically reported.

Sarilumab

Sarilumab (SAR) is a humanized monoclonal antibody, inhibiting the IL-6 receptor; it is approved for the treatment of adults with moderately to severely active RA. The rate of cardiovascular arrest reported in the EMA registry is relatively high (3.2%). Nevertheless, no specific data concerning QT prolongation and/or VAs in patients treated with SAR have been reported, and even a protective role (similar to TCZ) has been otherwise suggested, because of its immunomodulating effect, potentially decreasing the extent of myocardial injury frequently observed in COVID-19.[63] However, data in COVID-19 are scarce, and specific investigations on its effect on QT interval are lacking.

IL-1 inhibitors (anakinra and canakinumab)

Anakinra (ANA) and canakinumab (CAN) are the only 2 IL-1 inhibitors approved in Europe. Owing to the massive COVID-19 inflammatory reaction, it has been suggested that intravenous ANA and CAN could be used against the cytokine storm that seems to be associated with some extent of the lung damage in COVID-19. A metanalysis has shown that the administration of ANA in COVID-19 patients could be associated with reductions in both mortality and need for mechanical ventilation.[64] As for TCZ and SAR, specific data on the proarrhythmic or antiarrhythmic effect are lacking.

SUMMARY

Severe systemic inflammation and the off-label use of some drugs in COVID-19 may significantly prolong the QTc interval, potentially leading to a non-negligible risk of VAs. Among these drugs, CQ and HCQ have shown the higher risk of QTc prolongation and TdP, that is, however, overall low, even in association with other QT-prolonging drugs, such as AM.

In line with other authors,[65] also this panel believes that the ultimate aim of QTc surveillance during the COVID-19 pandemic should not result in an exclusion from potentially beneficial treatments or experimental clinic trials, but instead to identify patients at risk, in order to counterbalance and mitigate all potentially drug-induced arrhythmogenic side-effects.

CLINICS CARE POINTS

- Arrhythmic risk assessment is of pivotal importance when administering drug therapy in COVID-19.
- Several drugs may prolong QT interval in COVID-19, and particular attention should be paid to specific drugs combinations (e.g. chloroquine and hydroxychloroquine + macrolides).

REFERENCES

1. Gattinoni L, Coppola S, Cressoni M, et al. COVID-19 does not lead to a "typical" acute respiratory distress syndrome. Am J Respir Crit Care Med 2020;201(10):1299–300.
2. Busana M, Gasperetti A, Giosa L, et al. Prevalence and outcome of silent hypoxemia in COVID-19. Minerva Anestesiol 2021;87(3):325–33.
3. Zhou F, Yu T, Du R, et al. Clinical course and risk factors for mortality of adult inpatients with COVID-19 in Wuhan, China: a retrospective cohort study. Lancet 2020;395(10229):1054–62.
4. Wang D, Hu B, Hu C, et al. Clinical characteristics of 138 hospitalized patients with 2019 novel coronavirus-infected pneumonia in Wuhan, China. JAMA 2020;323(11):1061–9.
5. Huang C, Wang Y, Li X, et al. Clinical features of patients infected with 2019 novel coronavirus in Wuhan, China. Lancet 2020;395(10223):497–506.
6. Schiavone M, Gasperetti A, Mancone M, et al. Oral anticoagulation and clinical outcomes in COVID-19: an Italian multicenter experience. Int J Cardiol 2021;323:276–80.
7. Levi M, Thachil J, Iba T, et al. Coagulation abnormalities and thrombosis in patients with COVID-19. Lancet Haematol 2020;7(6):e438–40.
8. Ackermann M, Verleden SE, Kuehnel M, et al. Pulmonary vascular endothelialitis, thrombosis, and angiogenesis in Covid-19. N Engl J Med 2020; 383(2):120–8.
9. Schiavone M, Gasperetti A, Mancone M, et al. Redefining the prognostic value of high-sensitivity troponin in COVID-19 patients: the importance of concomitant coronary artery disease. J Clin Med 2020;9(10):3263.
10. Della Rocca DG, Magnocavallo M, Lavalle C, et al. Evidence of systemic endothelial injury and microthrombosis in hospitalized COVID-19 patients at different stages of the disease. J Thromb Thrombolysis 2021;51(3):571–6.
11. Shi S, Qin M, Shen B, et al. Association of cardiac injury with mortality in hospitalized patients with COVID-19 in Wuhan, China. JAMA Cardiol 2020; 5(7):802–10.
12. Wei JF, Huang FY, Xiong TY, et al. Acute myocardial injury is common in patients with COVID-19 and impairs their prognosis. Heart 2020;106(15):1154–9.
13. Lala A, Johnson KW, Januzzi JL, et al. Prevalence and impact of myocardial injury in patients hospitalized with COVID-19 infection. J Am Coll Cardiol 2020;76(5):533–46.
14. Schiavone M, Gobbi C, Biondi-Zoccai G, et al. Acute coronary syndromes and Covid-19: exploring the uncertainties. J Clin Med 2020;9(6):1683.
15. Li X, Guan B, Su T, et al. Impact of cardiovascular disease and cardiac injury on in-hospital mortality in patients with COVID-19: a systematic review and meta-analysis. Heart 2020;106(15):1142–7.
16. Mitacchione G, Schiavone M, Gasperetti A, et al. Ventricular tachycardia storm management in a COVID-19 patient: a case report. Eur Hear J Case Rep 2020;4(FI1):1–6.
17. Antwi-Amoabeng D, Beutler BD, Singh S, et al. Association between electrocardiographic features and mortality in COVID-19 patients. Ann Noninvasive Electrocardiol 2021. https://doi.org/10.111 anec.12833.
18. Romero J, Alviz I, Parides M, et al. T-wave inversion as a manifestation of COVID-19 infection: a case series. J Interv Card Electrophysiol 2020;59(3):485–9.
19. Tarighi P, Eftekhari S, Chizari M, et al. A review of potential suggested drugs for coronavirus disease (COVID-19) treatment. Eur J Pharmacol 2021;895: 173890.
20. Mitacchione G, Schiavone M, Curnis A, et al. Impact of prior statin use on clinical outcomes in COVID-19 patients: data from tertiary referral hospitals during COVID-19 pandemic in Italy. J Clin Lipidol 2021; 15(1):68–78.
21. Viskin S, Rosovski U, Sands AJ, et al. Inaccurate electrocardiographic interpretation of long QT: the majority of physicians cannot recognize a long QT when they see one. Heart Rhythm 2005;2(6):569–74.
22. Vandenberk B, Vandael E, Robyns T, et al. Which QT correction formulae to use for QT monitoring? J Am Heart Assoc 2016;5(6). https://doi.org/10.116 JAHA.116.003264.

3. Batchvarov VN, Ghuran A, Smetana P, et al. QT-RR relationship in healthy subjects exhibits substantial intersubject variability and high intrasubject stability. Am J Physiol Heart Circ Physiol 2002;282(6). https://doi.org/10.1152/ajpheart.00860.2001.

4. Postema PG, De Jong JSSG, Van der Bilt IAC, et al. Accurate electrocardiographic assessment of the QT interval: teach the tangent. Heart Rhythm 2008; 5(7):1015–8.

5. Postema PG, Arthur AMW. The measurement of the QT interval. Curr Cardiol Rev 2014;10(3):287–94.

6. Simpson TF, Salazar JW, Vittinghoff E, et al. Association of QT-prolonging medications with risk of autopsy-defined causes of sudden death. JAMA Intern Med 2020;180(5):698–706.

7. Schwartz PJ, Stramba-Badiale M, Crotti L, et al. Prevalence of the congenital long-qt syndrome. Circulation 2009;120(18):1761–7.

8. Moss AJ, Schwartz PJ, Crampton RS, et al. The long QT syndrome. Prospective longitudinal study of 328 families. Circulation 1991;84(3):1136–44.

9. Priori SG, Schwartz PJ, Napolitano C, et al. Risk stratification in the long-QT syndrome. N Engl J Med 2003;348(19):1866–74.

0. Nakano Y, Shimizu W. Genetics of long-QT syndrome. J Hum Genet 2016;61(1):51–5.

1. Schwartz PJ, Spazzolini C, Priori SG, et al. Who are the long-QT syndrome patients who receive an implantable cardioverter-defibrillator and what happens to them?: data from the European Long-QT syndrome implantable cardioverter-defibrillator (LQTS ICD) registry. Circulation 2010;122(13): 1272–82.

2. Forleo GB, Gasperetti A, Breitenstein A, et al. Subcutaneous implantable cardioverter defibrillator and defibrillation testing: a propensity-matched pilot study. Heart Rhythm 2021. https://doi.org/10.1016/j.hrthm.2021.06.1201.

3. Gasperetti A, Schiavone M, Ziacchi M, et al. Long term complications in patients implanted with subcutaneous implantable defibrillators Real-world data from the Extended ELISIR experience. Heart Rhythm 2021. https://doi.org/10.1016/j.hrthm.2021.07.008.

4. Lambiase PD, Eckardt L, Theuns DA, et al. Evaluation of subcutaneous implantable cardioverter-defibrillator performance in patients with ion channelopathies from the EFFORTLESS cohort and comparison with a meta-analysis of transvenous ICD outcomes. Heart Rhythm O2 2020;1(5):326–35.

5. Gasperetti A, Schiavone M, Ziacchi M, et al. Long-term complications in patients implanted with subcutaneous implantable cardioverter-defibrillators: real-world data from the extended ELISIR experience. Heart Rhythm 2021. https://doi.org/10.1016/j.hrthm.2021.07.008.

6. Schwartz PJ, Priori SG, Spazzolini C, et al. Genotype-phenotype correlation in the long-QT syndrome: gene-specific triggers for life-threatening arrhythmias. Circulation 2001;103(1): 89–95.

37. Moss AJ, Zareba W, Hall WJ, et al. Effectiveness and limitations of β-blocker therapy in congenital long-QT syndrome. Circulation 2000;101(6):616–23.

38. Tisdale JE, Jaynes HA, Kingery JR, et al. Development and validation of a risk score to predict QT interval prolongation in hospitalized patients. Circ Cardiovasc Qual Outcomes 2013;6(4):479–87.

39. Gasperetti A, Schiavone M, Tondo C, et al. QT interval monitoring and drugs management during COVID-19 pandemic. Curr Clin Pharmacol 2020;15. https://doi.org/10.2174/1574884715666201224155042.

40. Gao J, Tian Z, Yang X. Breakthrough: chloroquine phosphate has shown apparent efficacy in treatment of COVID-19 associated pneumonia in clinical studies. Biosci Trends 2020;14(1):72–3.

41. The RECOVERY Collaborative Group. Effect of hydroxychloroquine in hospitalized patients with Covid-19. N Engl J Med 2020;383(21):2030–40.

42. Reis G, Moreira Silva EADS, Medeiros Silva DC, et al. Effect of early treatment with hydroxychloroquine or lopinavir and ritonavir on risk of hospitalization among patients with COVID-19: the TOGETHER randomized clinical trial. JAMA Netw Open 2021; 4(4):e216468.

43. Ghazy RM, Almaghraby A, Shaaban R, et al. A systematic review and meta-analysis on chloroquine and hydroxychloroquine as monotherapy or combined with azithromycin in COVID-19 treatment. Sci Rep 2020;10(1):1–18.

44. Gasperetti A, Biffi M, Duru F, et al. Arrhythmic safety of hydroxychloroquine in COVID-19 patients from different clinical settings. Europace 2020;22(12): 1855–63.

45. Mazzanti A, Briani M, Kukavica D, et al. Association of hydroxychloroquine with QTc interval in patients with COVID-19. Circulation 2020;142(5):513–5.

46. Thémans P, Belkhir L, Dauby N, et al. Population pharmacokinetics of hydroxychloroquine in COVID-19 patients: implications for dose optimization. Eur J Drug Metab Pharmacokinet 2020;45(6):703–13.

47. Bernardini A, Ciconte G, Negro G, et al. Assessing QT interval in COVID-19 patients:safety of hydroxychloroquine-azithromycin combination regimen. Int J Cardiol 2021;324:242–8.

48. Chorin E, Wadhwani L, Magnani S, et al. QT interval prolongation and torsade de pointes in patients with COVID-19 treated with hydroxychloroquine/azithromycin. Heart Rhythm 2020;17(9):1425–33.

49. Cao B, Wang Y, Wen D, et al. A trial of lopinavir–ritonavir in adults hospitalized with severe Covid-19. N Engl J Med 2020;382(19):1787–99.

50. Owa AB, Owa OT. Lopinavir/ritonavir use in Covid-19 infection: is it completely non-beneficial? J Microbiol Immunol Infect 2020;53(5):674–5.

51. Haghjoo M, Golipra R, Kheirkhah J, et al. Effect of COVID-19 medications on corrected QT interval and induction of torsade de pointes: results of a multicenter national survey. Int J Clin Pract 2021; 75(7):e14182.

52. Mohanty S, Di Biase L, Mohanty P, et al. Effect of periprocedural amiodarone on procedure outcome in patients with longstanding persistent atrial fibrillation undergoing extended pulmonary vein antrum isolation: results from a randomized study (SPECULATE). Heart Rhythm 2015;12(3):477–83.

53. Zhu S, Wang J, Wang Y, et al. QTc prolongation during antiviral therapy in two COVID-19 patients. J Clin Pharm Ther 2020;45(5):1190–3.

54. Gupta AK, Parker BM, Priyadarshi V, et al. Cardiac adverse events with remdesivir in COVID-19 infection. Cureus 2020. https://doi.org/10.7759/cureus.11132.

55. Çap M, Bilge Ö, Işık F, et al. The effect of favipiravir on QTc interval in patients hospitalized with coronavirus disease 2019. J Electrocardiol 2020;63:115–9.

56. Çelik HG, Keske Ş, Şener Ü, et al. Why we should be more careful using hydroxychloroquine in influenza season during COVID-19 pandemic? Int J Infect Dis 2021;102:389–91.

57. Nakamura Y, Sasaki R, Cao X, et al. Intravenous anti-influenza drug oseltamivir will not induce torsade de pointes: evidences from proarrhythmia model and action-potential assay. J Pharmacol Sci 2016; 131(1):72–5.

58. Butler CC, Dorward J, Yu LM, et al. Azithromycin for community treatment of suspected COVID-19 in people at increased risk of an adverse clinical course in the UK (PRINCIPLE): a randomised,

controlled, open-label, adaptive platform trial. Lancet 2021;397(10279):1063–74.

59. Lazzerini PE, Acampa M, Capecchi PL, et al. Antiarrhythmic potential of anticytokine therapy in rheumatoid arthritis: tocilizumab reduces corrected QT interval by controlling systemic inflammation. Arthritis Care Res 2015;67(3):332–9.

60. Panoulas VF, Toms TE, Douglas KMJ, et al. Prolonged QTc interval predicts all-cause mortality in patients with rheumatoid arthritis: an association driven by high inflammatory burden. Rheumatol (Oxford) 2014;53(1):131–7.

61. Stone JH, Frigault MJ, Serling-Boyd NJ, et al. Efficacy of tocilizumab in patients hospitalized with Covid-19. N Engl J Med 2020;383(24):2333–44.

62. Rosas IO, Bräu N, Waters M, et al. Tocilizumab in hospitalized patients with severe Covid-19 pneumonia. N Engl J Med 2021;384(16):1503–16.

63. Lazzerini PE, Laghi-Pasini F, Acampa M, et al. IL-6 (interleukin 6) blockade and heart rate corrected QT interval prolongation in COVID-19. Circ Arrhythm Electrophysiol 2020;13(9):e008791.

64. Pasin L, Cavalli G, Navalesi P, et al. Anakinra for patients with COVID-19: a meta-analysis of non-randomized cohort studies. Eur J Intern Med 2021; 86:34–40.

65. Giudicessi JR, Noseworthy PA, Friedman PA, et al. Urgent guidance for navigating and circumventing the QTc-prolonging and torsadogenic potential of possible Pharmacotherapies for Coronavirus Disease 19 (COVID-19). Mayo Clin Proc 2020;95(6): 1213–21.

66. Drugs to be avoided by congenital long QT patients. Available at: www.crediblemeds.org. Accessed July 18, 2021.

Electrophysiology and Interventional Cardiology Procedure Volumes During the Coronavirus Disease 2019 Pandemic

Naga Venkata K. Pothineni, MD, Pasquale Santangeli, MD, PhD*

KEYWORDS

- Interventional cardiology • Electrophysiology • Procedures • Volume • COVID-19

KEY POINTS

- Volume of percutaneous coronary intervention has declined by >50% in the early phase of the pandemic across both North America and Europe.
- Largest decline in electrophysiology procedures was noted in elective catheter ablation procedures such as atrial fibrillation ablations.
- Universal preprocedural testing is an important part of safe resumption of elective procedures.
- Being prepared for further surges and waves of COVID is crucial for uninterrupted delivery of health care.

INTRODUCTION

The coronavirus disease 2019 (COVID-19) pandemic, caused by the severe acute respiratory syndrome coronavirus 2 (SARS-CoV-2), has imposed an unprecedented health care crisis across the globe. Health care efforts across the world have been diverted to tackling the pandemic since early 2020. Hospitals and health care systems have undertaken major restructuring in an effort to deliver health care to an increasing number of patients affected by COVID-19. Although great focus has been placed on treating those individuals suffering from COVID-19, clinicians must simultaneously balance caring for patients who are not actively infected. In anticipation of an exponential increase in COVID-19 cases, health care systems developed strategies to channel available resources to meet the rapidly rising demands of COVID-19. This change was noticed significantly in the field of invasive cardiology as well. Many cardiac catheterization and electrophysiology (EP) laboratories canceled elective procedures to limit the burden on hospital resources and preserve personal protective equipment (PPE). Major societies published guidance statements delineating patient selection for procedures during the exponential phase of the pandemic growth.[1] Patient care was triaged and those waiting for elective procedures were managed with expectant care or noninvasive approaches to preserve hospital resources and personnel. In the current article, we review the impact of the COVID-19 pandemic and its response to the volume of interventional cardiology (IC) and EP procedures across the world.

Funding Sources: None.
Section of Electrophysiology, Division of Cardiovascular Medicine, University of Pennsylvania, Philadelphia, PA, USA
* Corresponding author. Hospital of the University of Pennsylvania, 3400 Spruce Street, 9 Founders Pavilion, Philadelphia, PA 19104.
E-mail address: pasquale.santangeli@pennmedicine.upenn.edu

Card Electrophysiol Clin 14 (2022) 105–110
https://doi.org/10.1016/j.ccep.2021.10.011
1877-9182/22/© 2021 Elsevier Inc. All rights reserved.

Impact on Interventional Cardiology Procedures

Onset of the COVID-19 pandemic led to immediate cessation of multiple clinical services in the field of interventional cardiology for better resource allocation and avoidance of potential exposure, across various countries. The British Cardiovascular Interventional society conducted a retrospective study of all percutaneous coronary interventions (PCI) in the United Kingdom during the lockdown imposed by the pandemic and compared them to PCI volumes in the prepandemic period.[2] They showed that PCI volumes fell down by 49% with the greatest decrease in PCI for stable angina (66% reduction). PCI for ST-elevation MI (STEMI) was also down by 33%. Interestingly, the decline in volume was higher in older patients and in minorities. In another study from the United Kingdom, Mohamed and colleagues evaluated trends in all inpatient cardiac procedures to understand national trends during the lockdown period.[3] Data on interventional cardiac catheterization, PCI, electrophysiological (CIED implantation, catheter ablation), structural (TAVR), and surgical (CABG, SAVR, MVR) procedures were collected and compared with trends in preceding years. Overall procedural volume fell down by approximately 89% in April and May 2020 during the lockdown, with cardiac catheterization and CIED implantation being the most affected. In addition, after adjusting for baseline comorbidities, patients undergoing PCI, and CIED implantation in the lockdown period had higher odds of mortality. A 24% reduction (29% for NSTEMI and 18% for STEMI) in overall PCI volume for acute MI was also reported from a multicenter analysis from Ireland.[4]

Despite prioritization of STEMI care, when other interventional services were limited during the lockdown, a reduction was seen in STEMI activations and primary PCI procedures being performed, partly related to patient's reluctance to seek medical care during an ongoing pandemic. A single-center cross-sectional study from Germany reported a 50% reduction in admissions and primary PCI for acute MI during the early part of the pandemic than the prepandemic level.[5] More importantly, patients presenting with an acute MI during the pandemic had symptoms for a longer duration, presented with lower LV ejection fraction, had more immediate complications and 3 times higher mortality than the prepandemic levels. Similar results have been reported from other European countries such as Italy and Portugal.[6,7] A systematic review pooling data from 32 studies showed significantly prolonged door to balloon time and worse inpatient mortality for primary PCI for STEMI during the pandemic than prepandemic times.[8] To better understand STEMI care during the pandemic, multicenter registries were developed. The International Study of Acute Coronary Syndromes–ST-Elevation Myocardial Infarction (ISACS-STEMI) registry included data from 6609 patients that underwent primary PCI at 77 hospitals in 18 European countries.[9] There was a significant reduction in the volume of primary PCI in 2020 than in 2019, along with significantly longer door to balloon times and higher in-hospital mortality. The NACMI (North American COVID-19 and STEMI) prospective registry was developed to track STEMI management trends in patients with COVID-19.[10] This prospective multicenter study showed that patients with COVID-19 presenting with STEMI were less likely to receive primary PCI than controls and had higher rates of a composite of death, stroke, recurrent MI, and need for repeat revascularization.

Data on change in transcatheter aortic valve implantation volumes during the pandemic has been limited than studies evaluating PCI. Although experience from the United Kingdom showed no significant decline,[3] a survey from Asia showed 25% reduction in case of volume due to the pandemic.[11]

IMPACT ON ELECTROPHYSIOLOGY PROCEDURES

Response to the pandemic has also led to a reduction in EP procedures performed. During the surge of the pandemic, most EP programs only performed emergent procedures giving priority to ventricular tachycardia storms (ES), refractory device infections requiring lead/device extraction, urgent pacemaker and generator changes in PM-dependent patients A survey of 27 hospitals in the greater Philadelphia region evaluated the impact of COVID-19 on EP procedural volumes.[12] Data on procedural volumes in this study were generated from manufacturer sales records. This study showed that the onset of COVID-19 cases in the geographic region was associated with a reduction in both catheter ablation and device implantation procedures (Fig. 1). Monthly arrhythmia ablation procedures decreased by 88.4% from a bi-weekly baseline of 241 procedures before the onset of the US COVID-19 outbreak to 28 in late April 2020. Similarly, pacemaker and implantable cardioverter defibrillator procedures decreased by 74.4% (398–102 implants) over the same time interval.

Li and colleagues evaluated EP procedural volumes at three centers during a surge of COVID-19 in China, Italy, and United Kingdom.[13] In a

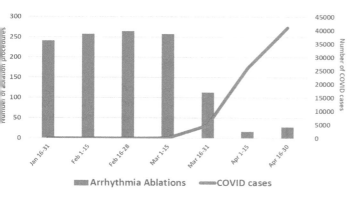

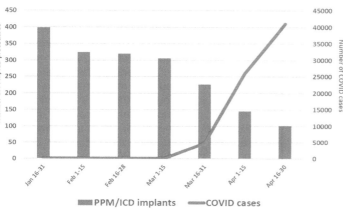

Fig. 1. Trends in EP procedural volumes in the greater Philadelphia region during the lockdown phase of the COVID-19 pandemic. (*From* Pothineni NVK, Santangeli P, Deo R, Marchlinski FE, Hyman MC. COVID-19 and electrophysiology procedures-review, reset, reboot!!!. J Interv Card Electrophysiol. 2020;59(2):303-305. https://doi.org/10.1007/s10840-020-00871-2; with permission)

hree centers, all elective EP procedures were canceled with an overall volume being less than ₀% of normal volumes. In addition, all EP ₍ersonnel were deployed for delivering emergency care out of EP. Arbelo and colleagues reported a ₊eduction in overall cardiac implantable electronic ₍evice (CIED) volumes in Spain as well during this ₍eriod.[14] In this study, data from 9 hospitals spanning 2017 to 2020 in the Catalonia province were ₊ggregated. Compared with the pre–COVID-19 ₍eriod, an absolute decrease of 56.5% was ₊bserved (54.7% in PM and 63.7% in ICD) in ₵IED implantation rates. Interestingly, there were ₊o statistically significant differences in the type ₊f PM or ICD implanted. An analysis of all cardiac ₍rocedures in the United Kingdom also revealed ₊n 89% and 56% reduction in catheter ablation ₊nd CIED implantation procedures in April 2020 ₊ompared with similar time periods in preceding ₊ears.[3] Similar reductions in CIED volumes from ₲ermany and Italy have been reported as well.[15,16]

₹ESUMPTION OF PROCEDURES – ₚRECAUTIONS AND UNIVERSAL TESTING

₊ollowing periods of lockdown in various ₊eographic regions, the resumption of elective procedures presented a challenge. Although measures to screen for symptomatic individuals for COVID-19 were widely available, the risk of asymptomatic carriers transmitting the infection to health care workers and other patients remained. Several infection control precautions were undertaken at many centers to combat this risk. As more tests became available, universal testing of patients had led to a safer resumption of elective services.

A prospective study of universal testing of all patients undergoing interventional and EP procedures has provided insight into a strategy of safe resumptions of elective procedures.[17] In this study conducted at the University of Pennsylvania, the following measures were instituted—universal surgical masks and temperature screening for all employees and patients, automated telephone preprocedure symptom screening for patients, strict restrictions on visitors for inpatients and outpatients, and universal preprocedure PCR testing to detect SARS-CoV-2 virus in patients undergoing elective or urgent procedures. Additional precautions to prevent cross-contamination were implemented at all feasible sites (**Table 1**). All inpatients undergoing cardiac catheterization or EP procedures underwent nasopharyngeal swabs

Table 1
Representative example of precautions in the interventional and electrophysiology laboratories during the resumption of elective cases

Risk	Proposed Measures
Coming and leaving in same scrubs	It is prohibited to come to work and leave with the same scrubs.
Common computer	Only work on personal laptops. Avoid sharing of computers (keyboards – difficult to clean)
Consent	Transition to verbal/e-consent
Contact	PPE as needed (gloves/mask)
Collecting PPE	Individualized packs
Lead aprons	Wipe and store in personal space
Control room equipment	Wipe Prucka before and after the case. Wear gloves to operate Prucka.
Anesthesia recovery	Wait in the control area, no computer work allowed
Provider contact	Limited provider contact unless absolutely necessary
Masking	All patients with masks in recovery and transfer
Break room	Limited to 2 people at a time for social distancing

for SARS-CoV-2 PCR testing performed at the hospital whereby the procedure was being performed. Outpatients were encouraged to undergo preprocedural testing at a satellite clinic 24 hours before the scheduled procedure to offload burden at the main hospital.

Over a study period of 1 month, a total of 215 patients underwent 252 elective or urgent procedures (128 catheterization and 124 EP procedures). 56% of procedures were performed on outpatients. Among 111 outpatients, 53 (47.7%) underwent testing at an off-site facility. All catheterization procedures were performed under moderate sedation; 30.6% of EP procedures were conducted under general anesthesia. Of 215 patients tested, 2 (0.9%) tested positive for SARS-CoV-2. No patients who tested negative at the time of their procedure subsequently tested positive for SARS-CoV-2, and no staff members developed any symptoms concerning COVID-19 during the universal testing period. During a follow-up telephone survey, two-thirds of patients reported that preprocedural testing did not change their

comfort level in getting the procedure performed and the rest reported increased comfort.

IMPACT ON TRAINEES

Not surprisingly, reduction in procedural volumes during the COVID-19 pandemic has impacted the training of fellows enrolled in interventional and EP training programs. Singla and colleagues conducted a survey of all EP fellows and program directors in the United States to assess the impact of the pandemic on EP training and education.[1] Out of 99 fellows that responded, 98% reported a decrease in their procedural volume and 55% of fellows reported a period of furlough or quarantine during the acute surge of COVID-19. A similar survey of 14 interventional cardiology programs in New York City also reported a significant reduction in catheterization procedures performed by fellows.[19] In this survey, more than two-thirds of interventional program directors opined that the pandemic has moderately to severely impacted fellowship training. 21% felt that fellows would graduate without performing 250 percutaneous coronary interventions (PCI), which is considered a minimum cut-off for graduation. A third of fellows and program directors felt that fellowship training should be extended to those impacted by the pandemic. Shah and colleagues conducted a larger survey through the Society for Cardiovascular Interventions and Angiography to which 133 interventional fellows responded.[20] By March 2020, only 43% of the respondents reported performing greater than 250 PCIs. With continued pandemic restrictions on elective procedures until the end of the fellowship, only 70% felt they would reach the minimum procedural volume cut-off for graduation. In addition to procedural volumes, trainees have also felt significant challenges due to the cancellation of in-person academic conferences and transition to purely web-based education. Job opportunities have dwindled down due to financial constraints imposed by the pandemic as well. Finally, the influence of the pandemic on fellow well-being cannot be ignored.[21]

FUTURE PREPAREDNESS

The development of a vaccine that is highly effective against moderate to severe COVID-19 has been a remarkable achievement. Increased vaccine uptake has led to a major reduction in hospitalizations for COVID-19 and enabled reopening to a state of near normalcy across the world. However, waves and surges of COVID-19 are expected to happen due to ongoing mutations in the virus and development of variants.[22] For instance, the current delta variant leading to surges in some parts of the United States has led to a rapid rise in hospitalizations again, overwhelming health care resources in some hospitals.[23] Although health care systems are more equipped to handle surges than the onset of the pandemic, these surges can lead to the cancellation of elective procedures again, impacting interventional and EP volumes as well. Lessons learnt from early 2020 can be used to better plan for effective and uninterrupted delivery of routine health care for chronic conditions, whereas handling the acute needs of an ongoing pandemic. There is no doubt that societal and governmental efforts to improve vaccine delivery and overall vaccination rates are pivotal to allow health care systems to effectively function.

CLINICS CARE POINTS

- Evaluation of local variations in COVID 19 cases and prioritization of resources should be implemented in anticipation of surges of infection.
- Remote monitoring of cardiac devices should be emphasized across all EP practices for better uninterrupted delivery of care in the event of further surges.
- Routine preprocedural testing and safety measures such as masking and encouraging vaccination should be routinely implemented until the pandemic resolves.
- Lessons learnt from the impact on procedures during the pandemic should be used for future planning.

DISCLOSURE

None related to this article.

REFERENCES

1. Lakkireddy DR, Chung MK, Gopinathannair R, et al. Guidance for cardiac electrophysiology during the COVID-19 pandemic from the Heart Rhythm Society COVID-19 Task Force; Electrophysiology Section of the American College of Cardiology; and the Electrocardiography and Arrhythmias Committee of the Council on Clinical Cardiology, American Heart Association. Circulation 2020 May 26;141(21):e823–31.
2. Kwok CS, Gale CP, Curzen N, et al. Impact of the COVID-19 pandemic on percutaneous coronary intervention in England: insights from the British Cardiovascular Intervention Society PCI Database Cohort. Circ Cardiovasc Interv 2020;13(11):e009654.
3. Mohamed MO, Banerjee A, Clarke S, et al. Impact of COVID-19 on cardiac procedure activity in England and associated 30-day mortality. Eur Heart J Qual Care Clin Outcomes 2021;7(3):247–56.
4. Connolly NP, Simpkin A, Mylotte D, et al. Impact on percutaneous coronary intervention for acute coronary syndromes during the COVID-19 outbreak in a non-overwhelmed European healthcare system: COVID-19 ACS-PCI experience in Ireland. BMJ Open 2021;11(4):e045590.
5. Primessnig U, Pieske BM, Sherif M. Increased mortality and worse cardiac outcome of acute myocardial infarction during the early COVID-19 pandemic. ESC Heart Fail 2021;8(1):333–43.
6. Azul Freitas A, Baptista R, Gonçalves V, et al. Impact of SARS-CoV-2 pandemic on ST-elevation myocardial infarction admissions and outcomes in a Portuguese primary percutaneous coronary intervention center: preliminary data. Rev Port Cardiol 2021;40(7):465–71.
7. D'Ascenzo F, De Filippo O, Borin A, et al. Impact of COVID-19 pandemic and infection on in hospital survival for patients presenting with acute coronary syndromes: a multicenter registry. Int J Cardiol 2021;332:227–34.
8. Chew NW, Ow ZGW, Teo VXY, et al. The global Effect of the COVID-19 pandemic on STEMI care: a systematic review and meta-analysis. Can J Cardiol 2021;37(9):1450–9. S0828-282X(21)00179-3.
9. De Luca G, Cercek M, Jensen LO, et al. Impact of COVID-19 pandemic and diabetes on mechanical reperfusion in patients with STEMI: insights from the ISACS STEMI COVID 19 Registry. Cardiovasc Diabetol 2020;19(1):215.
10. Garcia S, Dehghani P, Grines C, et al. Initial findings from the North American COVID-19 myocardial infarction registry. J Am Coll Cardiol 2021;77(16):1994–2003.
11. Tay EL, Hayashida K, Chen M, et al. Transcatheter aortic valve implantation during the COVID-19 pandemic: clinical expert opinion and consensus statement for Asia. J Card Surg 2020;35(9):2142–6.
12. Pothineni NVK, Santangeli P, Deo R, et al. COVID-19 and electrophysiology procedures-review, reset, reboot. J Interv Card Electrophysiol 2020;59(2):303–5.
13. Li J, Mazzone P, Leung LWM, et al. Electrophysiology in the time of coronavirus: coping with the great wave. Europace 2020;22(12):1841–7.
14. Arbelo E, Angera I, Trucco E, et al. Reduction in new cardiac electronic device implantations in Catalonia during COVID-19. Europace 2021;23(3):456–63.
15. Bollmann A, Hohenstein S, Meier-Hellmann A, et al. On behalf of Helios hospitals Group. Emergency hospital admissions and interventional treatments for heart failure and cardiac arrhythmias in Germany

during the Covid-19 outbreak: insights from the German-wide Helios hospital network. Eur Heart J Qual Care Clin Outcomes 2020;6:221–2.

16. Compagnucci P, Volpato G, Pascucci R, et al. Impact of the COVID-19 pandemic on a Tertiary-Level Electrophysiology Laboratory in Italy. Circ Arrhythm Electrophysiol 2020;13(9):e008774.

17. Pothineni NVK, Starkey S, Conn K, et al. Patient and staff perceptions of universal severe acute respiratory syndrome coronavirus 2 screening prior to cardiac catheterization and electrophysiology laboratory procedures. Circ Cardiovasc Interv 2020;13(12):e009975.

18. Singla VK, Jain S, Ganeshan R, et al. The impact of the COVID-19 pandemic on cardiac electrophysiology training: a survey study. J Cardiovasc Electrophysiol 2021;32(1):9–15.

19. Gupta T, Nazif TM, Vahl TP, et al. Impact of the COVID-19 pandemic on interventional cardiology fellowship training in the New York metropolitan area: a perspective from the United States epicenter. Catheter Cardiovasc Interv 2021;97(2): 201–5.

20. Shah S, Castro-Dominguez Y, Gupta T, et al. Impact of the COVID-19 pandemic on interventional cardiology training in the United States. Catheter Cardiovasc Interv 2020;96(5):997–1005.

21. Kadavath S, Hawwas D, Strobel A, et al. How the COVID-19 pandemic has affected cardiology fellow training. Am J Cardiol 2021;151:114–7.

22. Planas D, Veyer D, Baidaliuk A, et al. Reduced sensitivity of SARS-CoV-2 variant Delta to antibody neutralization. Nature 2021. https://doi.org/10.1038/s41586-021-03777-9.

23. Available at: https://www.wsj.com/articles/u-s-covid-19-hospitalizations-rise-as-delta-variant-spreads-11625780656. Accessed July 22, 2021.

Coronavirus Disease-19 Testing Strategies for Patients and Health Care Workers to Improve Workplace Safety

Sanghamitra Mohanty, MD, MS[a], Uriel Garcia, BS[b], Bryan MacDonald, MD[a],
Angel Mayedo, MD[a], Domenico G. Della Rocca, MD, PhD[a],
Carola Gianni, MD[a], Patrick Udenyi, BSc[c], William Zagrodzky, BS[a],
SaiShishir Shetty, DPharm, MHI[a], Andrea Natale, MD[a,d,e,*]

KEYWORDS

- COVID-19 • SARS-CoV-2 • Transmission • Viral shedding • Antibody assay • Viral antigen test
- Screening

KEY POINTS

- Universal testing at the workplace and subsequent home-isolation of identified cases successfully lowers the risk of horizontal transmission and creates a safe working environment
- In health care settings, close proximity while working and prolonged working hours make health care workers vulnerable to contracting the infection
- Presymptomatic and asymptomatic cases make it challenging to identify COVID-19 cases in the conventional symptom-based screening, reinforcing the usefulness of viral antigen, antibody, and RNA-based tests

Background: COVID-19 has been declared as a global health emergency with hundreds of millions being affected and many succumbed to this infectious disease since its first detection in China in December 2019.[1] Rapid emergence of mutant strains, high infection rate, and infection-mortality ratio coupled with limited knowledge about the severe acute respiratory syndrome coronavirus 2 (SARS-CoV-2) have made the management of this pandemic extremely challenging.[2] Subsequently, public health measures such as social distancing, universal use of facial masks, and restrictions at workplaces with shut-downs and lock-downs of many businesses have been imposed to limit the spread. However, the pandemic is far from being under control because of a continued surge of new variants and as a substantial share of the global population is still not immunized either due to their personal preferences or unavailability of the vaccine. Fearful patients suffering from other serious morbidities, with the intention of avoiding this highly contagious disease, reporting later in the disease progression resulting in poor outcome is another important collateral adversity of COVID-19.[2] Under this circumstance, with very little information to predict the course of this pandemic that has not yet shown any signs of remission, it is

[a] Texas Cardiac Arrhythmia Institute, St. David's Medical Center, Austin, TX, USA; [b] Universidad Anahuac, Mexico City, Mexico; [c] University of California - Berkeley, Berkeley, CA, USA; [d] Interventional Electrophysiology, Scripps Clinic, San Diego, CA, USA; [e] Metro Health Medical Center, Case Western Reserve University School of Medicine, Cleveland, OH, USA
* Corresponding author. 3000 North I-35, Suite 720, Austin, TX 78705.
E-mail address: dr.natale@gmail.com

Card Electrophysiol Clin 14 (2022) 111–114
https://doi.org/10.1016/j.ccep.2021.10.012
1877-9182/22/© 2021 Elsevier Inc. All rights reserved.

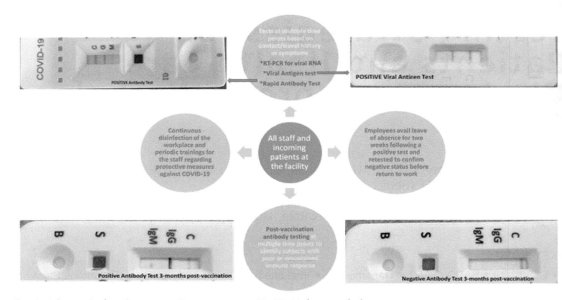

Fig. 1. Schematic showing strategies to create a COVID-19-free workplace.

highly crucial to find ways to create a safe environment for both patients and health care workers so that the health care institutions can continue providing the best care while protecting the health and wellbeing of all personnel involved and saving the community from the devastating toll of this pandemic on the economy and social fabric. This paper provides a brief overview of findings reported by different groups to mitigate workplace transmission of COVID-19.

Discussion: Viral shedding and transmission can happen in symptomatic as well as asymptomatic individuals infected with SARS-CoV-2 virus.[3] Shedding of replication-competent SARS-CoV-2 is believed to occur for 2 to 3 weeks following symptom onset and often much beyond the end of symptoms.[3] Moreover, presymptomatic and asymptomatic transmission can account for approximately 40%–45% of SARS-CoV-2 infections.[3] The characteristics of SARS-CoV-2 such as higher transmissibility, longer incubation period, asymptomatic transmission, and prolonged viral shedding illustrate the potential role of the workplace in SARS-CoV-2 transmission.[3] According to the Centers for Disease Control (CDC) guidelines, health care workers are at a very high risk for contracting this infection, which is not only while taking care of patients but most plausibly also by working closely with coworkers with unknown infection/contact status, for long hours.[4] In the beginning of the pandemic, of the 138 patients treated at Wuhan Hospital in China, 40 (29%) were health care workers.[4] Two systematic reviews reported up to 11% of the global

COVID-19 cases to be health care workers.[5] On prospective independent study documente health care workers in United Kingdom and Unite States to be at a significantly higher risk of con tracting the infection than the general population. Another trial by Schneider and colleagues demon strated multiple unprotected contacts betwee infected staff to be responsible for 4 outbreaks i their hospital.[7]

Because of the silent spread of this viral infec tion by asymptomatic and pre- and postsympto matic persons, besides vaccination, soci distancing and utilization of hygienic measures universal testing, screening, and surveillance ar highly critical in effectively identifying the sourc of infection and thus preventing horizontal trans mission in the target community.

In a multi-center study, we evaluated the eff cacy of widespread screening in creating a saf workplace in a consecutive series of 1670 asymp tomatic subjects (no symptoms of COVID-19 including patients and their caregivers and sta in our electrophysiology (EP) units.[2] Furthermore we assessed the new infection rate in patients un dergoing EP procedure, to see if identification an exclusion of positive cases facilitated the estab lishment of a risk-free operating environment.[2] A received serologic testing using COVID-19 Rapi Antibody Assays (Premier Biotech Labs, 72 Kasota Avenue SE, Minneapolis, MN 55414 an Confirm Biosciences, San Diego, CA) and naso pharyngeal (NP) swab was tested for viral RNA us ing ID NOW test kit from Abbott Diagnostics In (Scarborough, Maine). All test kits were cross verified internally by testing them against known COVID-19 positive and negative patients. Staff testing positive for viral-RNA on day 0 were asked for 2-week of self-isolation and were retested on day 14 before they got back to work. In 2 hospitals, personnel involved in patient care including technicians, nurses, physicians, dieticians, janitorial staff were retested at 14 to 21 days using an NP swab test for viral-RNA. Patients undergoing EP procedures were followed up for 2 weeks after being discharged from the hospital. They were asked to measure daily temperatures and report any symptoms of COVID-19 if experienced during the following 2-week period.

In our series, 64 (64/1670) cases tested positive for viral RNA at baseline, of which 33 were health care workers. All 33 staff members testing positive on day 0 were asked to self-quarantine for 2 weeks and were retested for viral RNA on day 14; 32/33 (96.9%) were negative and were allowed to get back to work. One staff with positive viral-RNA on day 14 tested negative on day 21 and returned to work then. None of the patients that received EP procedures during the study period reported symptoms of COVID-19 infection within 2 weeks after being discharged from the hospital.

A total of 67 patients were retested because of potential exposure to COVID-19 cases; 6 of the 67 tested positive. In these 6 positive cases, contact tracing revealed the possible source of infection to be family members or friends outside of the workplace. None of the coworkers of these 6 staff tested positive at that time.

As the findings demonstrate, universal testing and screening of all incoming patients, their caregivers, and hospital staff helped in identifying and isolating positive cases, thereby creating a safe working environment within the confines of our EP units.

In another observational study conducted in Wuhan, China, health screening (nucleic acid test for SARS-CoV-2, antibody detection, and chest CT scan) for COVID-19 was conducted among all returning staff from March to May 2020 that identified asymptomatic infection in some.[8] Close contacts of those positive cases were tracked, thereby curbing the risk of potential transmission at the workplace.[8]

Symptom screening before work entry is widely practiced in workplaces. However, high prevalence of asymptomatic illness attenuates the effectiveness of this strategy.[9] Haigh and colleagues reported the benefits of nonpharmaceutical interventions along with testing campaigns via reverse transcription-polymerase chain reaction (RT-PCR) of nasal swabs in late July to early August 2020, in 586 employees at 3 sites.[9] True positivity rates were consistent with community prevalence at the time; of all employees with positive tests, 99% were asymptomatic.[9] In a meta-analysis of 97 studies including 230,398 health care workers, estimated prevalence of SARS-CoV-2 infection was 11% and among the RT-PCR positive cases, 40% did not show symptoms at the time of diagnosis.[10]

As a high percentage of health care workers are vaccinated at this point and the overall epidemic wave is receding in countries, prospective patients should feel reassured about the low risk of contracting the infection in a health care setting. However, the risk still remains for those that are poor responders to COVID-19 vaccination or those that are unvaccinated. In an ongoing trial conducted by our group, ~85% of the staff were seen to have moderate to strong antibody (immunoglobulin G) response at 6 months following the second dose of COVID-19 vaccine (unpublished data). Thus, the antibody testing has also helped in identifying individuals lacking sustained immune response that could be vulnerable to future infection and would plausibly need booster doses for further protection.

These data reinforce the importance of multi-time point surveillance and screening of staff to create a COVID-19-free workplace in health care settings.[11]

Summary: Universal testing for COVID-19, at different time points as needed based on the contact history and/or symptoms would facilitate the prevention of horizontal transmission and creation of a safe workplace by identifying and isolating infectious cases. Given the continuing emergence of new viral strains with increased infectivity and severity and uncertainty of the efficacy of the available vaccines in providing protection against those new variants, the significance of widespread screening cannot be overemphasized while preparing workplaces worldwide for the safe return of employees and patients.

CLINICS CARE POINTS

To create a COVID-19-free workplace (**Fig. 1**).

- Employers should provide universal testing (RT-PCR for viral RNA, viral antigen, and antibody tests as deemed appropriate) facilities for all staff at multiple time points based on their travel/contact history and/or presenting symptoms

- Employees should consider taking leave of absence from work for 2 weeks after testing positive for viral antigen regardless of the symptom-status and repeat tests to confirm a negative result for COVID-19 before returning to work

- Vaccinations against COVID-19 should be highly recommended and antibody testing following vaccination should be performed at 3, 6, and 12 months to identify subjects with poor or unsustained immune response.
- Continuous disinfection of the workplace and periodic training for the staff regarding safety measures such as hand-washing, facial coverings, and timely reporting of their travel/contact history must diligently ensue

DISCLOSURES

Dr A. Natale is a consultant for Boston Scientific, Biosense Webster, St. Jude/Abbott Medical, Biotronik, Baylis, and Medtronic. Remaining authors have nothing relevant to disclose.

REFERENCES

1. Rueda-Garrido JC, Vicente-Herrero T, del Campo T, et al. Return to work guidelines for the COVID-19 pandemic. Occup Med 2020;70:300–5.
2. Mohanty S, Lakkireddy D, Trivedi C, et al. Creating a safe workplace by universal testing of SARS-CoV-2 infection in asymptomatic patients and healthcare workers in the electrophysiology units: a multi-center experience. J Interv Card Electrophysiol 2020;1–6. https://doi.org/10.1007/s10840-020-00886-9.
3. Plantes PJ, Fragala MS, Clarke C, et al. Model for mitigation of workplace transmission of COVID-19 through population-based testing and surveillance. Popul Health Manag 2021;24(S1):S16–25.
4. Rafeemanesh E, Ahmadi F, Memarzadeh M. A review of the strategies and studies on the prevention and control of the new Coronavirus in workplaces. Arch Bone Jt Surg 2020;8(Suppl1):242–6.
5. Sahu AK, Amrithanand VT, Mathew R, et al. COVID-19 in health care workers - a systematic review and meta-analysis. Am J Emerg Med 2020 Sep;38(9) 1727–31.
6. Nguyen LH, Drew DA, Joshi AD, et al. Risk of COVID-19 among frontline healthcare workers and the general community: a prospective cohort study medRxiv 2020. https://doi.org/10.1101/2020.04.29 20084111.
7. Schneider S, Piening B, Nouri-Pasovsky PA, et al. SARS-Coronavirus-2 cases in healthcare workers may not regularly originate from patient care: lessons from a university hospital on the underestimated risk of healthcare worker to healthcare worker transmission. Antimicrob Resist Infect Control 2020;9(1):192. https://doi.org/10.1186/s13756-020-00848-w.
8. Duan P, Deng ZQ, Pan ZY, et al. Safety considerations during return to work in the context of stable COVID-19 epidemic control: an analysis of health screening results of all returned staff from a hospital. Epidemiol Infect 2020;148:e214. https://doi.org/10.1017/S0950268820002150.
9. Haigh KZ, Gandhi M. COVID-19 mitigation with appropriate safety measures in an Essential workplace: lessons for Opening work settings in the United States during COVID-19. Open Forum Infect Dis 2021;8(4):ofab086. https://doi.org/10.1093/ofid/ofab086.
10. Gómez-Ochoa SA, Franco OH, Rojas LZ, et al. COVID-19 in health-care workers: a Living systematic review and meta-analysis of prevalence, risk Factors, Clinical characteristics, and outcomes. Am J Epidemiol 2021;190(1):161–75.
11. Treibel TA, Manisty C, Burton M, et al. COVID-19 PCR screening of asymptomatic health-care workers at London hospital. Lancet 2020 395(10237):1608–10.

Role of Digital Health During Coronavirus Disease 2019 Pandemic and Future Perspectives

Adnan Ahmed, MD[a], Rishi Charate, MD[a], Naga Venkata K. Pothineni, MD[a],
Surya Kiran Aedma, MD[b], Rakesh Gopinathannair, MD[a],
Dhanunjaya Lakkireddy, MD[a],*

KEYWORDS

- Digital health • Artificial intelligence (AI) • Machine learning (ML) • Deep learning (DL)
- COVID-19 pandemic • Telemedicine • Remote monitoring

KEY POINTS

- COVID-19 pandemic brought a significant paradigm shift in mode of health care delivery.
- Adoption of digital health served as a necessary tool to ensure safety of patients and health care professionals.
- Telemedicine, a concept that existed pre-COVID, was used to deliver care in outpatient as well as inpatient care settings to restrict exposure and conserve PPE.
- Barriers to wide-scale availability of digital health are related to lack of infrastructure, digital literacy, and patients belonging to underserved and underrepresented population with socioeconomic constraints.
- Economics of digital medical care and insurance reimbursements will continue to be a matter of debate in the near future.

INTRODUCTION

The coronavirus disease 19 (COVID-19) pandemic has yielded an unparalleled global challenge in the delivery of health care. From nationally mandated quarantines and mass vaccination efforts to ushering in a new era of virtual communication, it has necessitated a new perspective on health care moving forward. Specifically, it has led to institutionalized changes to health care systems, hospitals, medical professionals, ancillary staff, training programs, and health care polices. Aims to both safely preserve the best qualities of face-to-face traditional patient care as well as integrate technology and virtual care have been at the forefront of each specialty. Digital health care has been a revolution in this effort in effective management of patients with complex conditions. This paradigm shift has called for our advocacy to improve upon and incorporate even newer emerging digital health solutions as well as alleviate previous barriers to digital health care. Cardiac electrophysiology (EP) has been uniquely poised as a specialty that has been accustomed to using digital health techniques such as remote monitoring and artificial intelligence (AI) supplementary tools even in the prepandemic period.[1] In this article, we explain the obstacles encountered with in-person care during the pandemic, review currently available digital health platforms

[a] Kansas City Heart Rhythm Institute, 5100 W, 110th Street, Suite 200 Overland Park, KS 66211, USA; [b] Carle Foundation Hospital, 611 West Park Street, Urbana, IL 61801, USA
* Corresponding author. Kansas City Heart Rhythm Institute, 5100 W, 110th Street, Suite 200, Overland Park, KS 66211, USA.
E-mail address: dhanunjaya.lakkireddy@hcahealthcare.com

Card Electrophysiol Clin 14 (2022) 115–123
https://doi.org/10.1016/j.ccep.2021.10.013

specifically in relation to cardiac EP, and explore further avenues for advancing digital and in-person care delivery in the future.

TRADITIONAL CARE DURING THE PANDEMIC

The COVID-19 pandemic has abruptly ushered in a foundational change to the traditional practice of medicine. Despite clinical research and advancements continually evolving and reshaping the field of medicine, the practice of face-to-face patient encounters had previously remained stable. Although face-to-face care was accepted as the norm for centuries, the pandemic forced us to revisit this idea as a community. This pandemic was the catalyst for not only a sudden but also a widespread paradigm shift in patient care, with nearly 80% of the US population indicating that they have used one form of digital health.[2,3] The pandemic has also enabled health care providers and administrators to revisit the intricacies of in-person care delivery and improve overall efficiency. In-person care depends on a variety of supporting frameworks that include providers, administrative personnel, patients, caregivers, and family members and is very time and resource intensive. Testing for COVID-19 and limiting physical contact between personnel for in-person care made for a more complex, time-consuming, and inefficient process. One study advocated for creating a safe workplace by universal testing for COVID-19 in asymptomatic patients and health care workers. Out of 1670 subjects, 758 were patients and 912 were caregivers, Emergency Medical Service, and EP laboratory personnel. The study found 3.8% positivity rates in the asymptomatic population.[4] While hospitals began cancellation of elective clinic and procedural visits in efforts to allocate health care resources toward tackling the pandemic, a steep decline in patient comfort levels in attending in-person visits was also noted. Several reports have indicated patient hesitancy to attend for in-person care even for concerning anginal symptoms. In fact, there was a reduction in patients presenting to the emergency room with acute myocardial infarction during the peak of the pandemic, and those that presented had higher mechanical complications due to late presentations.[5] These data highlight the hesitancy and overt concern that patients may have to seek medical care in this current global crisis, which can sometimes be life threatening. Cardiac EP has also seen a decline in in-person visits across the globe during the pandemic. However, EP has an advantage of decision making being driven by abstract data such as rhythm monitors, electrocardiograms, and device interrogations, which enabled a smoother transi-tion to virtual care.

DIGITAL HEALTH IN ELECTROPHYSIOLOGY DURING CORONAVIRUS DISEASE 2019
Remote Monitoring

Cardiac EP has been a leader in digital health care. Over the years multitude of devices have been developed and implemented in clinical practice, and these services were increasingly used during the pandemic in addition to development of some novel tools. Remote cardiac monitoring can be classified into 3 broad categories:[1]

- Medical-grade wearable monitors such as Holter monitor and external and internal loop recorder.
- Consumer-grade wearable monitors such as smartwatches.
- Cardiac implantable electronic devices (CIEDs) such as pacemakers and defibrillators.

These diverse range of devices generate different types of data. Holter and loop recorders only function as data collectors, whereas CIEDs can recognize critical findings and intervene based on programming. As a result, remote monitoring bears a prognostic value and helps in reducing worse outcomes. CIEDs received a class I recommendation for remote monitoring in 2015.[6] However, in the prepandemic times remote monitoring was underused due to patient- and system-based issues. The pandemic made remote monitoring an important tool to help identify critical and noncritical issues and address them accordingly. Enrollment of existing patients in device clinics in remote monitoring was an important initiative undertaken by various EP programs in response to the pandemic.[8] One Italian study reported an experience of 332 patients introduced to remote monitoring during the lockdown. Patients were categorized based on modality, divided between remote monitoring at home versus office. Study findings reported high patient satisfaction, and providers were better able to provide continuous health care coverage in eligible CIED patients.[9]

Remote monitoring enables informed triage of patients needing urgent procedures, clinical decision making and diagnosis, and implementation of appropriate therapeutic interventions while bypassing an in-person visit. Similarly, patients adopting digital health tools like pulse oximeters, automated blood pressure equipment, glucose monitors, and single-lead electrocardiograph (ECG) recorders were able to provide their respective physicians with important data without risking exposure.

One important aspect of remote monitoring is the burden of data received and the challenge of trained personnel being available to accurately review and act upon the data. Development of novel AI tools that can incorporate machine learning (ML) can help stratify the findings, so that appropriate measures can be taken.[1]

The concept of drive-through pacing clinics fills the gap for the subset of patients who may not be suitable for remote monitoring. This familiar concept involved patients driving up parallel to a kiosk occupied by a health care worker. A study by Akhtar and colleagues[10] evaluated 316 patients of which 66.8% had pacemakers, 21.8% had cardiac resynchronization therapy (CRT) devices, and 1.1% had implantable cardioverter-defibrillators. A total of 50 wound inspections were performed, and 2 were diagnosed and treated for superficial infections. Seven were diagnosed with new-onset atrial fibrillation (AF) and were referred for anticoagulation. Device settings were adjusted in 6.1% of cases, and only 22 patients were referred to a physician for a variety of symptoms. Most patients (57.1%) preferred this drive-through format over the conventional methods.[10]

Telemedicine

The concept of telemedicine existed in the pre-COVID era, but it was limited and often complicated with reimbursement issues for physicians. The COVID-19 crisis led to rapid adoptions of virtual medical care. At present telemedicine is provided by telephones, secure messaging, and audio-video conference calls via commercial applications. The Office for Civil Right expressed willingness to forego penalties for Health Insurance Portability and Accountability Act noncompliance among providers enacting in good faith measures for telemedicine during the pandemic.[11]

In an attempt to conserve personal protective equipment (PPE), avoid exposure for patients and clinicians, and limit both hospitalizations for non-COVID reasons and outpatient office visits, an array of tele-health care was provided to patients in inpatient and outpatient settings. The Heart Rhythm Society (HRS)/American college of cardiology (ACC)/American Heart Association (AHA) provided an early guidance for electrophysiologists on how to practice during the pandemic. The guidance advocated for virtual visits, emphasizing social distancing, conservation of PPE, and minimizing face-to-face encounters when possible; it also clearly addressed nonurgent/nonemergent procedures, protocols for performing procedures on patients with COVID-19.[12]

Berman and colleagues[13] shared their experience of managing 29 inpatient EP consultations at the heart of the pandemic in New York. The investigators were able to manage 55% of patients remotely and were able to provide guideline- and evidence-based recommendations.[13] Similar reports came from other specialties like OB/GYN in which they were able to provide telehealth to 1352 patients for prenatal care, of which 61.5% were maternal-fetal medicine visits.[14] Another pilot study was reported by Renner and colleagues[15] from Helsinki University Hospital in Finland. The investigators performed 25 tele-rounds in 15 patients in the pulmonary ward; they concluded that tele-rounding is feasible in select patients with COVID-19 and can improve health care workers' safety and conserve PPE.[15]

Whether the current exponential growth in telemedicine will continue to grow after the pandemic is over is yet to be seen. However, with mass-scale vaccinations being delivered globally and humanity seeking a return to normalcy, we do believe the unexpected outcome of COVID-19 is reliance upon digital health, which can be seen in forms like physical fitness, adherence to therapies, ordering medications, and disease screening tools as part of smartphone/tablet apps.

We hypothesize that these adoptions may improve patient satisfaction, avoid long wait times in offices, avoid travel, and discuss medical care at the comfort of their homes. A study by Han and colleagues[3] reported that 60% of patients and 70% of clinicians would prefer to continue with virtual telehealth visits in future. This concept will also aid busy specialist physicians who tend to cover multiple hospitals to make recommendations via digital visits, improve recommendation times, and eventually improve hospital length of stay.

Artificial Intelligence Tools

AI has been incorporated into medicine for some decades now, but its incorporation to modern day clinical practice is reaching new horizons with the start of the COVID 19 pandemic. AI refers to machine-based processing of data that typically requires human cognitive function. ML is a subgroup of AI that uses algorithms to learn patterns empirically from data; it identifies nonlinear relationships and higher-order interactions between multiple variables, which are often difficult to obtain via traditional statistics. Deep learning (DL) is a powerful ML approach that analyzes large complex data sets and enables efficient decisions. AI tools have brought about significant change in cardiac EP and cardiovascular imaging as well. AI has shown promise in assisting in diagnosis, disease prediction models, and response to treatment and prognosis.[16]

The concept of AI is not new in cardiac EP with automated ECG interpretations existing since the 1970s.[17] However, interpretation of ECGs relies on expert opinion and requires training and expertise. Algorithms for the computerized automated diagnosis of 12-lead ECGs in prehospital setting can really aid emergency medical personnel or nonspecialist physicians to identify a condition and timely start treatment in high-risk patients. However, current automated ECG diagnosis algorithms lack accuracy and result in misdiagnosis if not reviewed carefully. There has been substantial progress in these areas where ECG-based deep neural networks (DNNs) have been tested to identify arrhythmias, classify supraventricular tachycardias, and predict left ventricular hypertrophy. A study by Attia and colleagues,[18] which included 180,922 patients, in which AI-enabled ECG during normal sinus rhythm was able to identify AF with almost 80% accuracy. Another good example is the study by Ko and colleagues in which they used a trained and validated convolutional neural network using 12-lead ECG and were able to detect hypertrophic cardiomyopathy with a sensitivity up to 95%. We do believe that these DNN models require more refinement and validation but in future are likely to aid specialists and nonspecialists with improved ECG diagnosis and perhaps as screening tools.[19–22]

Other dimensions related to ECGs are the use of implantable devices, smartwatches, and smartphone-based apps, which can generate large amounts of data sets that are not amenable for manual evaluation. Arrhythmia detection algorithms on DNNs on large sets of ambulatory patients with single-lead plethysmography have shown similar diagnostic performance as cardiologists and implantable loop recorders. Continuous monitoring provides the opportunity to pick up asymptomatic cardiac arrhythmias and overcome serious adverse events in future.[21]

Electroanatomic mapping in complex invasive EP procedures provides another opportunity. By combining data from diagnostic tools like MRI and fluoroscopy, previous electroanatomical mapping can help identify arrhythmogenic substrates and decrease the invasive catheter ablation times. There has been development in integrating fluoroscopy and electroanatomical mapping with MRI with ML.[23,24]

The above-mentioned examples provide a framework of tools in AI, but their wide-scale validation and translation into clinical practice may not be that far away.

Electrophysiology-Specific Innovations

Some examples of EP-specific innovations are described in the following sections.

Tele-atrial fibrillation project

AF is the most common cardiac arrhythmia; its traditional management requires face-to-face evaluations with cardiologist and primary care doctors and checking heart rate (HR) and rhythm control with ECG. With lockdowns and health facilities under pressure, telehealth visits became the backbone for providing care. However, effective management is limited in patients with AF because it did not allow for measurements of HR or checking the rhythm during the telehealth visit. To overcome this and make a unified structure all over Europe, The Cardiology Department of the Maastricht University Medical Center+ (MUMC+) in Maastricht, the Netherlands, innovated a standard operating procedure document describing the TeleCheck-AF approach. This approach involved teleconsultation coupled with remote photoplethysmography-based HR and heart rhythm monitoring (FibriCheckVR) to allow the treating clinicians to manage their patient comprehensively. FibriCheckVR currently enroll 2492 patients in about 40 clinical centers around Europe. Patients once enrolled are requested to check their HR and heart rhythm via the application twice a day for at least 7 days before doctor's visit. The physician evaluates the rhythms in real time and reports it in a user-friendly dashboard. Further changes in clinical management will be addressed by physicians via teleconsultations.

This is a great example in which varying infrastructure in different countries were able to set up the concept of mobile health (mHealth) in a short duration of time. FibriCheckVR was easy to use and install by patients. Further prospective trials are underway to assess if mHealth is noninferior to current standard care guided by face-to-face consultations.[2,25]

Smartphone electrocardiographic surveillance

Another great example in this association is the use of smartphone for ECG surveillance to preserve hospital capacity during the pandemic. The idea was to empower primary care physicians and patients with appropriate tools to identify patients with concerns for clinical deterioration with stable COVID-19 infection. The study involved 2 primary care physicians who enrolled 521 patients. The physicians were equipped with 8/12-lead hospital-grade smartphone-operated ECG device (D-Heart). First ECG was done under the supervision of the physician, and they were instructed to record at least one ECG at day 4 of infection o whenever cardiac symptoms were present during the first 10 days of infection. ECG was evaluated 24/7 within 15 minutes of arrival via telecardiology platform by cardiologists. This is reported to be the first study of its kind and enabled primary care physicians for early detection and avoiding a worse clinical outcome. The study concluded that the smartphone-controlled ECG devices are ideal for simple arrhythmia assessments but may not be adequate for complex ECG evaluation.[26] Certainly, this methodology lays a nice platform for multiparametric telemonitoring for patients in the future with improvement and acceptability of telehealth.

Home antiarrhythmic drug loading with smartphone tracings

Outpatient loading of antiarrhythmic drugs (AAD) like sotalol and dofetilide has been a matter of debate. Although outpatient initiation of sotalol is approved in certain cases, clinicians prefer to admit patients and monitor them closely for QT interval prolongation and development of ventricular arrhythmias. As COVID-19 stretched the health care systems all over the world, it led to delays in hospitalization for initiation of AAD and elective ablation procedures to help ensure maintenance of sinus rhythm versus rate control strategy. These circumstances led to the initiative of starting these medications in outpatient setting with patients who had CIEDs. Two separate studies by Mascarenhas and colleagues[27,28] for dofetilide (n = 30 patients) and sotalol (105 patients) demonstrated that they were able to successfully initiate these medications in the outpatient setting with careful telemonitoring. In both studies Permament Pace makers and Intra-cardiac defibrillators were programmed to provide a lower rate of pacing at 70 bpm and Implantable loop recorders were programmed to detect an HR greater than 150 to 160 bpm depending on the device used. A mandatory 2-hour manual transmission was obtained after initiation of medication. Patients were seen in office for the first 3 days of initiation of medication.[27,28]

Although larger cohorts may be needed to validate these findings, these studies do lay a good foundation and direction for future studies. This outpatient initiative not only decreases the risk of nosocomial infections, including COVID-19, but also helps to decrease the cost burden by avoiding hospitalization of 3 days.

Heart logic

CRT devices have now been incorporated in multiple studies with ML to predict end points like heart failure or death after CRT by using multitude of baseline variables. Heart Logic is a good example of a personalized, remote heart failure diagnostic and monitoring solution and has been validated to provide weeks of advance notice for early signs of worsening heart failure.[29]

The ML models have outperformed current guidelines in predicting response and improved event-free survivals, although these findings are modest at this time. In other reports ML has been able to predict mortality better than preexisting clinical risk scores.[30,31]

BARRIERS TO DIGITAL HEALTH DELIVERY

Virtual care and digital health were instrumental in care delivery during the pandemic. Cancellation of elective procedures and visits was the immediate response, whereas creation of alternative digital solutions such as virtual telemedicine visits and remote patient monitoring measures represented a long-term viable strategy.[7] However, this transition was far from seamless and posed significant difficulties during its immediate implementation. First, the resource burden from the COVID-19 pandemic required a prioritization of essential procedures, and with this in mind a return to full force in the postpandemic period can place additional strain on digital health care delivery given that it continues to be evolving in terms of familiarity and efficiency.[32] Furthermore, the sheer volume of data inflow that can be expected with CIEDs, both medical- and consumer-grade wearable monitors, and incorporated AI tools can be overwhelming. This burden of increased data can present challenges to incorporation into clinical practice and can be overwhelming once in-person care returns to full volumes. Additional quality control parameters are needed because the accuracy of some of these devices is still precocious.[1] Along with this data influx, an efficient and accurate triaging system must be in place, and AI tools, although improving, still lack this ability reliably.[1] In a comparative prepandemic and peripandemic survey regarding the changes in the digital health landscape among cardiac EP professionals, the most common barrier cited was a lack of infrastructure, which despite showing an improvement between the 2 surveys still remained a prominent problem even after reassessment and highlights the lag of a supportive framework despite advancements in digital health.[3] This fact must be taken into consideration with the reintegration of face-to-face encounters, and with the progression of digital health moving forward. Our familiarity with digital health and its limits is still expanding, although more specifically this puts us as providers in the impactful role to ensure digital literacy to our patients.[33] Although smartphone applications, digital wearable devices, and virtual telemedicine appointments have served to further patient care, this comes with a learning curve for the user itself and makes providers the fulcrum of digital literacy education and patient advocacy in this area. Furthermore, these digital health solutions also serve both themselves as social barriers to health and can further highlight already present health care disparities.[3] Digital health usually requires access to Wi-Fi, Bluetooth, and/or smartphones, which may not be routinely available to all patients. Patients in underserved or underrepresented populations and with socioeconomic barriers are experiencing a compounded gap in care.[34] Specifically, a multivariate analysis consisting of 148,402 patients who had either completed or missed telemedicine appointments revealed that age greater than 55 years, Asian ethnicity, Medicaid insurance care, and non-English-speaking patients were most vulnerable to the digital divergence in care.[35] African American and Latinx communities with household incomes of less than $50,000 had lower rates of video telemedicine visits compared with telephone visits, which could limit some of the offered video conference benefits such as medication reconciliations or virtual physical examinations.[35] The demand, therefore, for more applications of digital health must also be met with equal support for digital health equity, an equally vital social disparity in the current state of medicine.[34] Finally, a virtual move to collective educational platforms such as national and global health conferences has remained a topic of discussion, with some claiming its potential to reach a wider audience yet others highlighting the inability to provide hands-on experience, and interdisciplinary learning.[32] As vaccination efforts continue to curb the impact of the pandemic, and in-person patient care has been slowly reintegrating, resurgences can halt this process, and the supplementary role of digital health must be continually reevaluated. Finding a steady state in which overreliance is not placed upon digital health while still using these resources to extract as much patient data to complement face-to-face interactions is paramount.

Fig. 1 summarizes the flow of digital health in clinical cardiac EP.

DIGITAL HEALTH IN THE POSTPANDEMIC PERIOD

Two main overarching factors will outline the future of digital health: digital health infrastructure and government policies for reimbursement.[3] Economics remains a fundamental driver for impacting changes in medical care. The Centers for Medicare and Medicaid have responded with basic billing code implementation and addition for telemedicine to encompass a wide spectrum and acuity of patient encounters, and it remains to be seen if other insurance carriers will follow this pathway as well as if this continues to be fostered and expanded in the future.[1,32]

Other improvements have come in the form of applicability and accessibility. The utilization of learning models such as Project ECHO (Extension of Community Healthcare Outcomes) is a collaborative multispecialty videoconferencing program that aims to promote peer-to-peer multidisciplinary learning to health care providers as well as make them comfortable as a technology provider in the digital health landscape.[3] Furthermore, the advocacy seen from organizations such as Telehealth for Seniors, Inc, a Florida-based nonprofit organization aiding in provision of digital health devices and education for seniors, has emerged during the pandemic as well as increases in telehealth platform funding from the Coronavirus Aid, Relief, and Economic Security (CARES) Act[3,37]; these have contributed to the increase in accessibility to digital health although these gaps in digital health disparity have not been bridged and advocacy for digital health equity must remain pressured.[34] Successful continued advocacy and resultant expansion of digital health can hope to present new telemedicine models to more remote areas and reach a wider spectrum of patients.

A further application of digital health in the future postpandemic period will hope to focus on the impact of digital health on clinical research and namely, its recruitment. Predating the COVID-19 pandemic, efforts such as the MyHeart Counts and Heart eHealth studies used app-based recruitment and wearable monitoring devices to create larger cohorts and easier, prolonged periods of study.[38] Pairing this with the advancements necessitated in digital health, there is an optimistic outlook on the contribution of digital health tools in patient recruitment and ease of monitoring to contribute to higher cohorts in clinical research.

EP serves as a fertile foundation for the incorporation of AI, and the ideal role it plays in the future is still budding. The hope for AI to assist in triaging and risk stratification in various cardiac disease provides for an enticing outlook, and it can be hoped that these advancements will continue to be cultivated, as their application currently remains limited.

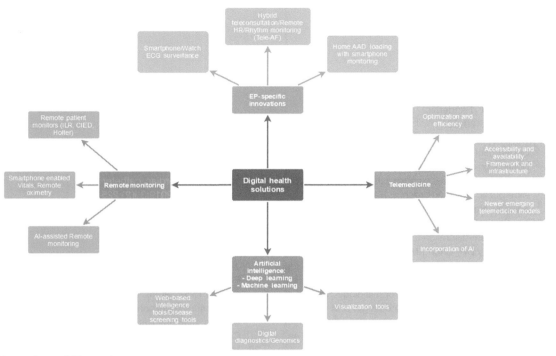

Fig. 1. Central illustration.

SUMMARY

New digital health innovations and an accommodating digital health landscape have shown promise during this pandemic, and we find ourselves as a field faced with the challenge of continuing to cultivate and incorporate this aspect of medicine. Consumer-grade wearable monitors, AI triaging and diagnostic supplementary tools, and improved accessibility to technology mark some of the foreseen changes to the field of cardiac EP. This knowledge will allow us to focus on restructuring the comprehensive and traditional albeit resource-intensive in-person model of patient care, and we hope to transition to a more efficient, patient-centered, and communicative framework both incorporating digital health and reincorporating in-person care moving forward.

REFERENCES

1. Slotwiner DJ, Al-Khatib SM. Digital health in electrophysiology and the COVID-19 global pandemic. Heart Rhythm O2 2020;1(5):385–9.
2. Gawalko M, Duncker D, Manninger M, et al. The European TeleCheck-AF project on remote app-based management of atrial fibrillation during the COVID-19 pandemic: centre and patient experiences. Europace 2021;23(7):1003–15.
3. Han JK, Al-Khatib SM, Albert CM. Changes in the digital health landscape in cardiac electrophysiology: a pre-and peri-pandemic COVID-19 era survey. Cardiovasc Digit Health J 2021;2(1):55–62.
4. Mohanty S, Lakkireddy D, Trivedi C, et al. Creating a safe workplace by universal testing of SARS-CoV-2 infection in asymptomatic patients and healthcare workers in the electrophysiology units: a multicenter experience. J Interv Card Electrophysiol 2020;62(1):171–6.
5. Primessnig U, Pieske BM, Sherif M. Increased mortality and worse cardiac outcome of acute myocardial infarction during the early COVID-19 pandemic. ESC Heart Fail 2021;8(1):333–43.
6. Slotwiner D, Varma N, Akar JG, et al. HRS Expert Consensus Statement on remote interrogation and monitoring for cardiovascular implantable electronic devices. Heart Rhythm 2015;12(7):e69–100.
7. Lakkireddy DR, Chung MK, Deering TF, et al. Guidance for rebooting electrophysiology through the COVID-19 pandemic from the Heart Rhythm Society and the American Heart Association Electrocardiography and Arrhythmias Committee of the Council on Clinical Cardiology: Endorsed by the American College of Cardiology. Circ Arrhythm Electrophysiol 2020;13(7):e008999.
8. Pothineni NVK, Santangeli P, Deo R, et al. COVID-19 and electrophysiology procedures-review, reset, reboot!!! J Interv Card Electrophysiol 2020;59(2):303–5.

9. Piro A, Magnocavallo M, Della Rocca DG, et al. Management of cardiac implantable electronic device follow-up in COVID-19 pandemic: lessons learned during Italian lockdown. J Cardiovasc Electrophysiol 2020;31(11):2814–23.

10. Akhtar Z, Montalbano N, Leung LWM, et al. Drive-Through Pacing Clinic: A Popular Response to the COVID-19 Pandemic. JACC Clin Electrophysiol 2021;7(1):128–30.

11. enforcement, U.S.D.o.H.H.S.H.g.N.o., et al., U.S. Department of Health & Human Services. HHS.gov. Notification of enforcement for discretion for telehealth remote communications during the COVID-19 nationwide public health emergency. March 30, 2020. Available at: https://www.hhs.gov/hipaa/for-professionals/special-topics/emergency-preparedness/notification-enforcement-discretion-telehealth/index.html.

12. Lakkireddy DR, Chung MK, Gopinathannair R, et al. Guidance for cardiac electrophysiology during the COVID-19 pandemic from the Heart Rhythm Society COVID-19 task force; Electrophysiology Section of the American College of Cardiology; and the Electrocardiography and Arrhythmias Committee of the Council on Clinical Cardiology, American Heart Association. Heart Rhythm 2020;17(9):e233–41.

13. Berman JP, Abrams MP, Kushnir A, et al. Cardiac electrophysiology consultative experience at the epicenter of the COVID-19 pandemic in the United States. Indian Pacing Electrophysiol J 2020;20(6):250–6.

14. Madden N, Emeruwa UN, Friedman AM, et al. Telehealth uptake into prenatal care and provider attitudes during the COVID-19 pandemic in New York City: a quantitative and qualitative analysis. Am J Perinatol 2020;37(10):1005–14.

15. Renner A, Paajanen J, Reijula J. Tele-rounding in a university hospital pulmonary ward during the COVID-19 pandemic: a pilot study. Infect Dis (Lond) 2020;52(9):669–70.

16. Feeny AK, Chung MK, Madabhushi A, et al. Artificial intelligence and machine learning in arrhythmias and cardiac electrophysiology. Circ Arrhythm Electrophysiol 2020;13(8):e007952.

17. Nygårds ME, Hulting J. An automated system for ECG monitoring. Comput Biomed Res 1979;12(2):181–202.

18. Attia ZI, Noseworthy PA, Lopez-Jimenez F, et al. An artificial intelligence-enabled ECG algorithm for the identification of patients with atrial fibrillation during sinus rhythm: a retrospective analysis of outcome prediction. Lancet 2019;394(10201):861–7.

19. Hannun AY, Rajpurkar P, Haghpanahi M, et al. Cardiologist-level arrhythmia detection and classification in ambulatory electrocardiograms using a deep neural network. Nat Med 2019;25(1):65–9.

20. Perlman O, Katz A, Amit G, et al. Supraventricular tachycardia classification in the 12-lead ECG using atrial waves detection and a clinically based tree

21. van de Leur RR, Boonstra MJ, Bagheri A, et al. Big data and artificial intelligence: opportunities and threats in electrophysiology. Arrhythm Electrophysiol Rev 2020;9(3):146–54.

22. Ko WY, Siontis KC, Attia ZI, et al. Detection of hypertrophic cardiomyopathy using a convolutional neural network-enabled electrocardiogram. J Am Coll Cardiol 2020;75(7):722–33.

23. van Es R, van den Broek HT, van der Naald M, et al. Validation of a novel stand-alone software tool for image guided cardiac catheter therapy. Int J Cardiovasc Imaging 2019;35(2):225–35.

24. van den Broek HT, Wenker S, van de Leur R, et al. 3D Myocardial Scar Prediction Model Derived from Multimodality Analysis of Electromechanical Mapping and Magnetic Resonance Imaging. J Cardiovasc Transl Res 2019;12(6):517–27.

25. Pluymaekers NAHA, Hermans ANL, van der Velden RMJ, et al. On-demand app-based rate and rhythm monitoring to manage atrial fibrillation through teleconsultations during COVID-19. Int J Cardiol Heart Vasc 2020;28:100533.

26. Maurizi N., Fumagalli C., Cecchi F., et al. 202 ztab009. Published 2021 Jan 29. Use of Smartphone operated ECG for home ECG surveillance in COVID-19 patients. 2021. https://doi.org/10.1093/ehjdh/ztab009.

27. Mascarenhas DAN, Mudumbi PC, Kantharia BK. Outpatient initiation of dofetilide: insights from the complexities of atrial fibrillation management during the COVID-19 lockdown. J Interv Card Electrophysiol 2021;1–8. https://doi.org/10.1007/s10840-021-00942-y.

28. Mascarenhas DAN, Mudumbi PC, Kantharia BK. Outpatient initiation of sotalol in patients with atrial fibrillation: utility of cardiac implantable electronic devices for therapy monitoring. Am J Cardiovasc Drugs 2021;1–8. https://doi.org/10.1007/s40256-021-00493-7.

29. Gardner RS, Singh JP, Stancak B, et al. HeartLogic Multisensor Algorithm Identifies Patients During Periods of Significantly Increased Risk of Heart Failure Events: Results From the MultiSENSE Study. Circ Heart Fail 2018;11(7):e004669.

30. Feeny AK, Rickard J, Patel D, et al. Machine learning prediction of response to cardiac resynchronization therapy: improvement versus current guidelines. Circ Arrhythm Electrophysiol 2019;12(7):e007316.

31. Hu SY, Santus E, Forsyth AW, et al. Can machine learning improve patient selection for cardiac resynchronization therapy? PLoS One 2019;14(10):e0222397.

32. Alkhouli M, Coylewright M, Holmes DR. Will the COVID-19 Epidemic reshape cardiology? Eur Heart J Qual Care Clin Outcomes 2020;6(3):217–20.

scheme. IEEE J Biomed Health Inform 2016;20(6):1513–20.

3. Cowie MR, Lam CSP. Remote monitoring and digital health tools in CVD management. Nat Rev Cardiol 2021;18(7):457–8.

4. Crawford A, Serhal E. Digital health equity and COVID-19: The innovation curve cannot reinforce the social gradient of health. J Med Internet Res 2020;22(6):e19361.

5. Eberly LA, Kallan MJ, Julien HM, et al. Patient characteristics associated with telemedicine access for primary and specialty ambulatory care during the COVID-19 pandemic for primary and specialty ambulatory care during the COVID-19 pandemic. JAMA Netw Open 2020;3(12):e2031640.

36. Hunt RC, Struminger BB, Redd JT, et al. Virtual peer-to-peer learning to enhance and accelerate the health system response to COVID-19: The HHS ASPR Project ECHO COVID-19 Clinical Rounds Initiative. Ann Emerg Med 2021;78(2):223–8.

37. Verma A. 2020. Available at: https://www.telehealthforseniors.org/contact. Accessed July 30, 2021; TeleHealth Access for Seniors, Inc.

38. Sharma A, Harrington RA, McClellan MB, et al. Using digital health technology to better generate evidence and deliver evidence-based care. J Am Coll Cardiol 2018;71(23):2680–90.

Impact of COVID-19 Pandemic on Cardiac Electronic Device Management and Role of Remote Monitoring

Michele Magnocavallo, MD[a,b], Giampaolo Vetta, MD[a],
Alessia Bernardini, MD[a], Agostino Piro, MD[a], Maria Chiara Mei, MD[a],
Martina Di Iorio, MD[a], Marco Valerio Mariani, MD[a],
Domenico G. Della Rocca, MD, PhD[b], Paolo Severino, MD, PhD[a],
Raffaele Quaglione, MD[a], Giuseppe Giunta, MD[a],
Cristina Chimenti, MD, PhD[a], Fabio Miraldi, MD[a], Carmine Dario Vizza, MD[a],
Francesco Fedele, MD[a], Carlo Lavalle, MD[a,*]

KEYWORDS

- COVID-19 • Remote monitoring • Telemedicine • CIED • Telehealth • Pacemaker
- Implantable cardiac defibrillator

KEY POINTS

- The aim of remote monitoring is to optimize the clinical management of CIED patients, improve quality of life, and reduce hospitalization and emergency department access.
- A well-established organizational model should include an adequately structured team, a valid integration with the primary health care centers, and an appropriate response to clinical alerts.
- The development and refinement of telemedicine during the pandemic period suggest that remote monitoring should be recommended for all CIED patients.

INTRODUCTION

On December 31, 2019, a cluster of pneumonia cases of unknown origin was reported in the city of Wuhan; severe acute respiratory syndrome coronavirus 2 (SARS-CoV-2) was then discovered as the causative agent of the respiratory disease named coronavirus disease 2019 (COVID-19).[1] The epidemic spread rapidly through China and subsequently to the rest of the world, leading the World Health Organization to declare the pandemic state on March 11, 2020.

COVID-19 has caused a global impact on public health services that led to the reorganization of hospital settings, including in-office visits for patients with cardiac implantable electronic device (CIED). Remote monitoring (RM) of CIED patients represents an appropriate strategy to minimize any potential risk of virus exposure for patients and health care providers, without compromising the quality of care.[2–5] RM offers access to the same information as an in-office visit and may contribute to the early detection of atrial and ventricular arrhythmias,[6,7] prevent heart failure (HF) decompensation, and manage device-related issues.[8–12] RM has also confirmed its usefulness in decreasing the hospitalization rate and improving clinical outcomes.[13] Moreover, since the onset of the COVID-19 pandemic, physicians have suspended nonurgent scheduled visits and made a rapid transition to virtual visits (VV).[14–16] Thanks

a Department of Cardiovascular/Respiratory Diseases, Nephrology, Anesthesiology, and Geriatric Sciences, Policlinico Umberto I, Sapienza University of Rome, Rome, Italy; b Texas Cardiac Arrhythmia Institute, St. David's Medical Center, 3000 North IH-35, Suite 720, Austin, TX 78705, USA
* Corresponding author.
E-mail address: carlolavalle@uniroma1.it

Card Electrophysiol Clin 14 (2022) 125–131
https://doi.org/10.1016/j.ccep.2021.10.010
1877-9182/22/© 2021 Elsevier Inc. All rights reserved.

to the technological improvement, patients utilizing wearable sensors for the measurement of hemodynamic parameters (blood pressure and saturation, heart rate) and adopting virtual health platforms may be monitored directly from home without any risk of infection.

In this review, we provide an overview of the many possible applications of RM, its limitations and challenges in patients with CIED during the COVID-19 pandemic.

THE ROLE OF RM IN CIED MANAGEMENT DURING COVID-19

RM of CIED patients has become increasingly popular in clinical practice, especially during the COVID-19 pandemic.[17] Indeed, in the new guidelines of the European Society of Cardiology (ESC) on cardiac pacing, RM is recommended to reduce the number of in-office follow-up in patients with pacemaker (PMK) who have difficulties to attend in-person visits. RM may also be useful in case of a device component that has been recalled or is on advisory, to enable early detection of actionable events in patients at high risk.[18] RM provides the same information as an in-person visit ensuring an early identification of cardiac arrhythmias, such as ventricular tachycardias or atrial fibrillation, device therapy, and device-related issues like lead malfunction and early battery discharge.[19–22] Additional benefits were also demonstrated among HF patients in terms of preventing unfavorable cardiovascular events and reducing hospital readmissions.[12,23]

Although guidelines recommended the use of RM for the follow-up of patients with CIED, the coverage of RM was limited because of the organizational problems of health care systems and reimbursement issues.[18,20] The COVID-19 pandemic forced all health care providers to minimize interpersonal contacts to limit the spread of the virus, which led to a total reshaping of outpatient cardiology management and accelerated the deployment and widespread use of RM.[24] Indeed, the consensus document of the Heart Rhythm Society (HRS) and ESC for the management of cardiovascular disease during the COVID-19 pandemic recommended that RM should replace in-office visits for device interrogation and, whenever possible, postpone the scheduled in-person visit.[3,4,14,24,25]

A questionnaire-based survey by the European Heart Rhythm Association (EHRA) to assess the influence of the COVID-19 pandemic on RM in CIEDs demonstrated a strong implementation of RM in patients with PMKs and implantable loop recorders (ILRs; PMK 24.2 vs 39.9%; $P = .002$; ILR

61.5 vs 73.5%; $P = .028$). A nonsignificant increasing trend was registered for RM of cardiac resynchronization therapy-pacemaker (CRT-P devices (44.5 vs 55%; $P = .063$), implantable cardioverter defibrillators (ICDs; 65.2 vs 69.6% $P = .408$) and CRT-defibrillators (CRT-D; 65.2 v 68.8%; $P = .513$).[26]

Home delivery of the transmitter for RM should be preferred over in-office delivery, as it limit the exposure of patients to the hospital environment. To date, home delivery of transmitter i feasible for Boston Scientific and Abbott PM and ICDs, as well as for the latest Medtronic CIED with BlueSync.[24] As demonstrated in a recent multicenter study, the communicator LATITUDE was home delivered to 1324 patients from 4 different Italian centers and successful activatio through telephone training was achieved in 92% of cases.[27] Moreover, De Larochellière and colleagues confirmed that switching from a follow up model with in-person visits to an RM mode did not impair the management of ICD patients and significantly reduced the number of in person visits.[28] In **Fig. 1**, we summarized a protocol for setting up and managing RM during th COVID-19 pandemic. When the device is suitabl for RM, home delivery of the transmitter is a appropriate strategy for minimizing any potentia risk of virus exposure for patients and healt care providers.

Overall, the available evidence confirmed tha RM is an easy-to-use and effective tool for th management of CIED patients even during th pandemic and demonstrated that the home deliv ery and activation of communicators without an in patient visit is a potential opportunity to furthe extend RM in the future.

SUPPLEMENTATION OF TELECONSULTATION IN CIED PATIENTS

The ESC and HRS consensus documents stated that in-person visits should be replaced by tele medicine consultations in order to prevent th spread of the virus among cardiovascular pa tients.[3,24] Indeed, the worldwide survey by Ha and colleagues about the use of eHealth technolo gies during the COVID-19 pandemic showed a sig nificant increase in the use of teleconsultations i the management of cardiological patients (5.9% vs 58.6%; $P < .001$) for all types of consultation compared with the prepandemic period.[25]

Supplementing teleconsultation in CIED pa tients could be a key tool in the management c these patients during the COVID-19 pandemic especially for those affected by HF. ICD and CR have the capability of monitoring HF by measurin

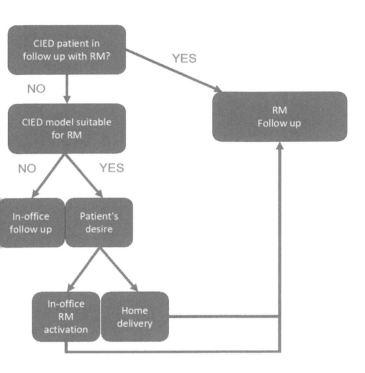

Fig. 1. Remote monitoring setup protocol. CIED, cardiac implantable electronic device; RM, remote monitoring.

noracic impedance (Optivol, Medtronic; CorVue, Abbott)[29] or by integration of several indices HeartLogic, Boston Scientific).[30] Nevertheless, guidance statements issued by experts in electrophysiology and HF recommend that every effort should be made to convert in-office visits to telehealth and VV. Specifically, the VVs used for decades to reach remote communities,[31] but less commonly used in advanced health care systems, have now emerged as the cornerstone of ambulatory care in all subspecialties.[32] The potential benefits of VV for HF patients are providing access to care and medical advice, which would be otherwise difficult to obtain and reducing in-person exposure to SARS-CoV-2. Cardiac rhythm professionals are advantaged by having wireless technology available to transmit monitored information to keep them connected.[33] Moreover, VVs have the advantage of detecting and alerting caregivers about relevant parameter changes, allowing earlier hospitalization of the patient, even in a presymptomatic phase.[34] A flowchart for VV is summarized in **Fig. 2**; VV was recommended in patients with atrial arrhythmias, alert for HF decompensation and nonsustained ventricular tachycardia.

Overall, new technologies and digital platforms to aid in remote care should be developed and further research on the role of telehealth, continuous data collecting, advanced automotive features, and RM is needed to guide best practices.

PATIENT ACCEPTABILITY AND SATISFACTION OF RM DURING COVID-19

As in any health care interaction, patient involvement plays an important role, and in the case of RM, active participation is fundamental. Patients must adhere to transmission timetables and keep in contact with the physician to guarantee a successful health care system based on RM. Therefore, from a positive reciprocal interaction between patient and caregiver usually derives a high acceptability and satisfaction. From the point of view of the patient, especially during the COVID-19 period, RM should be ease of use,[35–37] even when manual transmission of the data is requested, and guarantee a positive relationship with their health care provider at enrollment and during all the monitored period.[36,38–40] The Home Monitoring Acceptance and Satisfaction Questionnaire is administered to evaluate the acceptability and satisfaction of RM (HoMASQ) and showed that ICD patients had a higher level of acceptance and satisfaction than patients with PMK.[35,39] Moreover, RM was demonstrated to be easy to use and well accepted even for older people and patients with a low level of scholarity.[41] Otherwise, the most frequent causes of noncompliance seem to be:

- age-related: age under 40 years was associated with lower compliance.

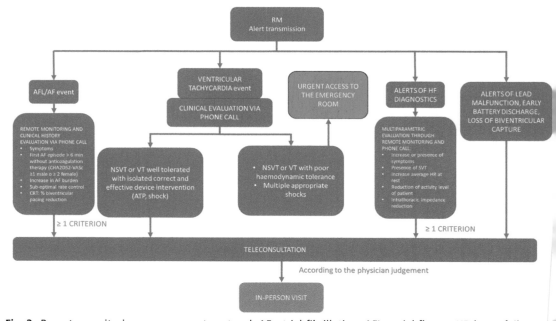

Fig. 2. Remote monitoring management protocol. AF, atrial fibrillation; AFL, atrial flutter; HF, heart failure; HR, heart rate; NSVT, non-sustained ventricular tachycardia; RM, remote monitoring; SVT, supraventricular tachycardia; VT, ventricular tachycardia.

- Health care systems–related: high volume clinics were associated with better compliance.
- Device-related: wireless devices are characterized by a better compliance compared with those requiring use of a wand.[42]

The institution of an RM patient agreement supported by the HRS enhances the compliance because patients can freely share information and experiences.[17]

During the COVID-19 pandemic, also the delivery of the communicator for RM could reduce the risk of contagion and influence patient's acceptability. Piro and colleagues demonstrated that home delivery of the communicator and intensive transtelephonic support for its activation resulted in an easy understanding of the device activation process, as well as high satisfaction with the use of the transmitter.[2] In addition, despite the ongoing pandemic and national lockdown, patients referred a sense of security and expressed interest in continuing with RM; also, in-office modem delivery and activation was associated with a higher prevalence of anxiety symptoms due to COVID-19 pandemic, compared with home modem delivery.[2,27]

In conclusion, several studies showed a high level of patient satisfaction and compliance, making it possible to extend this form of management

to a growing volume of patients, especially in times of pandemics.

RM FOR CIED PATIENTS WITH OTHER COMORBIDITIES

CIED patients are usually affected by multiple comorbidities: neurologic syndromes, chronic kidney disease, chronic obstructive pulmonary disease, diabetes mellitus, and other endocrinological disorders. New technologies and the adaptation of existing telemedicine tools represent an alternative option for an integrated monitoring.[3,32] For example, diabetes patients need recurrent medical consultations to optimize drug therapy and blood sugar levels, and telemedicine can be a valuable alternative, especially during a pandemic when contacts need to be limited.[43] To confirm the effectiveness of RM for diabetes management, a recent meta-analysis demonstrated a reduction in glycated hemoglobin in the RM group compared with controls.[44] Moreover, continuous glucose monitoring is effective in the management of high-risk patients with type 1 diabetes mellitus without any diabetic ketoacidosis.[45]

Telemedicine also spread into the field of neurology and a telestroke unit was established to allow remote assessment of patients with suspected stroke to minimize unnecessary in-person visits.[46] The latest evidence demonstrated that in-hospital management of end-stage renal disease patients increased the risk of infection up to 4 times compared with telemedicine-based home management and was more expensive. Similarly, RM appeared effective in the rehabilitation and management of chronic obstructive pulmonary disease patients, leading to a reduction in hospitalizations and emergency department visits.[47]

All this evidence shows how the pandemic escalated the adoption of telemedicine and all aspects of digital health, and this new reality is now likely to define medicine in the future not only in cardiology but also in other branches of medicine.

ECONOMIC ASPECTS

In addition to primary analyses focusing on cardiovascular outcomes (hospitalizations, cardiovascular death, overall death), another important aspect to consider for the adoption of digital health solutions is their impact on health care expenditure.[48,49] Owing to the outbreak of the SARS-CoV-2, a prompt reorganization of health care services was necessary with a related new economic-financial business plan.

The TARIFF study demonstrated that the overall mean annual cost per patient for in-office follow-up was significantly higher than an RM-based one (−53.87% in the RM group). The main reason for cost reduction is due to the cost of cardiovascular hospitalizations (€ 886.67 ± €1979.13 vs €432.34 ± €2488.10; P = .0030).[50] The same findings were reported in the EVOLVO study, a multicenter clinical trial aiming at measuring the benefits of RM for HF patients with ICDs. The results of this study showed that RM was cost-effective with an average saving of €888.10 per patient.[48] Notably, cost-effectiveness between countries varied considerably depending on whether there was specific reimbursement for RM services. In fact, there was heterogeneity among countries, with RM generating less profits for providers in the absence of specific reimbursements and similar or increased profits in cases such reimbursements existed.[51] Indeed, according to a recent European survey, the absence of reimbursement in many countries is generally considered the major barrier to the implementation of RM in standard practice.[20]

RM was cost-effective for health care systems because of lower follow-up costs and hospitalization reductions; the future challenge will be a more uniform deployment of appropriate reimbursement systems.

SUMMARY

The COVID-19 pandemic imposed challenges to the traditional rules of access and delivery of health care worldwide.[52] It accelerated the adoption of telemedicine and digital health, confirming a new era in the management of CIED patients. Patient outcomes could be improved with device-based intensive monitoring compared with traditional in-clinic follow-up at regular intervals.[53] The pandemic experience promoted the search for alternative solutions for an effective patient follow-up, such as validation of digital technologies, data management strategies, implementation of predictive analytics, cybersecurity, development of limited forms of remote CIED programming, and reimbursement.[19,51,54]

CLINICS CARE POINTS

- Remote Monitoring should be proposed in all CIED patients.
- Remote Monitoring is safe and effective also during COVID pandemic.
- Virtual Visit might be used in patients with multiple cardiac comorbidities.

DISCLOSURES

The authors have nothing to disclose.

REFERENCES

1. Zhu N, Zhang D, Wang W, et al. A novel Coronavirus from patients with pneumonia in China, 2019. N Engl J Med 2020;382:727–33.
2. Piro A, Magnocavallo M, Della Rocca DG, et al. Management of cardiac implantable electronic device follow-up in COVID-19 pandemic: lessons learned during Italian lockdown. J Cardiovasc Electrophysiol 2020;31:2814–23.
3. Varma N, Marrouche NF, Aguinaga L, et al. HRS/EHRA/APHRS/LAHRS/ACC/AHA worldwide practice update for telehealth and arrhythmia monitoring during and after a pandemic. EP Europace 2021;23:313.
4. Mohanty S, Lakkireddy D, Trivedi C, et al. Creating a safe workplace by universal testing of SARS-CoV-2 infection in asymptomatic patients and healthcare workers in the electrophysiology units: a multi-center experience. J Interv Card Electrophysiol 2020. https://doi.org/10.1007/s10840-020-00886-9.
5. Della Rocca DG, Magnocavallo M, Lavalle C, et al. Evidence of systemic endothelial injury and

microthrombosis in hospitalized COVID-19 patients at different stages of the disease. J Thromb Thrombolysis 2020. https://doi.org/10.1007/s11239-020-02330-1.

6. Della Rocca DG, Santini L, Forleo GB, et al. Novel perspectives on arrhythmia-induced cardiomyopathy: pathophysiology, clinical manifestations and an update on invasive management strategies. Cardiol Rev 2015;23:135–41.

7. Chen Q, Xu J, Gianni C, et al. Simple electrocardiographic criteria for rapid identification of wide qrs complex tachycardia: the new limb lead algorithm. Heart Rhythm 2020;17:431–8.

8. Forleo GB, Panattoni G, Schirripa V, et al. Device monitoring of heart failure in cardiac resynchronization therapy device recipients: a single-center experience with a novel multivector impedance monitoring system. J Cardiovasc Med 2013;14:726–32.

9. Ong MK, Romano PS, Edgington S, et al. Effectiveness of remote patient monitoring after discharge of hospitalized patients with heart failure: the better effectiveness after transition–heart failure (BEAT-HF) randomized clinical trial. JAMA Intern Med 2016;176:310.

10. García-Fernández FJ, Osca Asensi J, Romero R, et al. Safety and efficiency of a common and simplified protocol for pacemaker and defibrillator surveillance based on remote monitoring only: a long-term randomized trial (RM-ALONE). Eur Heart J 2019;40:1837–46.

11. Pignalberi C, Mariani MV, Castro A, et al. Sporadic high pacing and Shock impedance on remote monitoring in Hybrid implantable cardioverter-Defibrillator systems: clinical impact and management. Heart Rhythm 2021;18:1292–300.

12. Boehmer JP, Hariharan R, Devecchi FG, et al. A multisensor algorithm predicts heart failure events in patients with implanted devices. JACC: Heart Fail 2017;5:216–25.

13. Hindricks G, Taborsky M, Glikson M, et al. Implant-based multiparameter telemonitoring of patients with heart failure (IN-TIME): a Randomised Controlled trial. Lancet 2014;384:583–90.

14. AIAC Ricerca Network Investigators, Boriani G, Palmisano P, Guerra F, et al. Impact of COVID-19 pandemic on the clinical activities related to arrhythmias and electrophysiology in Italy: results of a survey promoted by AIAC (Italian association of arrhythmology and cardiac pacing). Intern Emerg Med 2020;15:1445–56.

15. Hollander JE, Carr BG. Virtually perfect? Telemedicine for covid-19. N Engl J Med 2020;382:1679–81.

16. Lakkireddy DR, Chung MK, Gopinathannair R, et al. Guidance for cardiac electrophysiology during the COVID-19 pandemic from the heart rhythm Society COVID-19 Task Force; electrophysiology section of the American College of cardiology; and the Electrocardiography and arrhythmias Committee of the Council on clinical cardiology, American heart association. Heart Rhythm 2020;17:e233–41.

17. Slotwiner D, Varma N, Akar JG, et al. HRS expert consensus statement on remote interrogation and monitoring for cardiovascular implantable electronic devices. Heart Rhythm 2015;12:e69–100.

18. Glikson M, Nielsen JC, Kronborg MB, et al. ESC guidelines on cardiac pacing and cardiac resynchronization therapy. Eur Heart J 2021;2021:ehab364.

19. Saxon LA, Varma N, Epstein LM, et al. Factors influencing the decision to proceed to firmware upgrades to implanted pacemakers for cybersecurity risk mitigation. Circulation 2018;138:1274–6.

20. Mairesse GH, Braunschweig F, Klersy K, et al. Implementation and reimbursement of remote monitoring for cardiac implantable electronic devices in Europe: a survey from the health economics Committee of the European heart rhythm association. EP Europace 2015;17:814–8.

21. Della Rocca Domenico G, Albanese M, Placidi F, et al. Feasibility of automated detection of sleep apnea using implantable pacemakers and defibrillators: a comparison with simultaneous polysomnography recording. J Interv Card Electrophysiol 2019;56:327–33.

22. Forleo GB, Tesauro M, Panattoni G, et al. Impact of continuous intracardiac st-segment monitoring on mid-term outcomes of ICD-Implanted patients with coronary artery disease. Early results of a prospective comparison with conventional ICD outcomes. Heart 2012;98:402–7.

23. Dang S, Dimmick S, Kelkar G. Evaluating the evidence Base for the Use of home telehealth remote monitoring in Elderly with heart failure. Telemedicine e-Health 2009;15:783–96.

24. The European Society for Cardiology. ESC Guidance for the Diagnosis and Management of CV Disease during the COVID-19 Pandemic. Available at: https://www.escardio.org/Education/COVID-19-and-Cardiology.

25. Han JK, Al-Khatib SM, Albert CM. Changes in the digital health landscape in cardiac electrophysiology: a pre-and peri-pandemic COVID-19 era survey. Cardiovasc Digital Health J 2021;2:55–62.

26. Simovic S, Providencia R, Barra S, et al. The use of remote monitoring of cardiac implantable devices during the COVID-19 pandemic: an EHRA physician survey. EP Europace 2021. https://doi.org/10.1093/europace/euab215. euab215.

27. Magnocavallo M, Bernardini A, Mariani MV, et al. Home delivery of the communicator for remote monitoring of cardiac implantable devices: a multicenter experience during the Covid-19 lockdown. Pacing Clin Electrophysiol 2021;44:995–1003.

38. De Larochellière H, Champagne J, Sarrazin J-F, et al. Findings of remote monitoring of implantable cardioverter defibrillators during the COVID-19 pandemic. Pacing Clin Electrophysiol 2020;43:1366–72.

39. Abraham WT, Compton S, Haas G, et al. Intrathoracic impedance vs daily weight monitoring for predicting worsening heart failure events: results of the fluid accumulation status trial (FAST). Congest Heart Fail 2011;17:51–5.

40. Boehmer JP, Hariharan R, Devecchi FG, et al. A multisensor algorithm predicts heart failure events in patients with implanted devices: results from the MultiSENSE study. JACC Heart Fail 2017;5:216–25.

41. Bagchi S. Telemedicine in Rural India. Plos Med 2006;3:e82.

42. Sayed S. COVID-19 and diabetes; possible role of polymorphism and rise of telemedicine. Prim Care Diabetes 2021;15:4–9.

43. Steinberg JS, Varma N, Cygankiewicz I, et al. 2017 ISHNE-HRS expert consensus statement on ambulatory ECG and External cardiac monitoring/telemetry. Heart Rhythm 2017;14:e55–96.

44. Varma N, Epstein AE, Irimpen A, et al. TRUST investigators efficacy and safety of automatic remote monitoring for implantable cardioverter-defibrillator follow-up: the lumos-t safely reduces routine office device follow-up (TRUST) trial. Circulation 2010; 122:325–32.

45. Morichelli L, Porfili A, Quarta L, et al. Implantable cardioverter defibrillator remote monitoring is well Accepted and easy to use during long-Term follow-up. J Interv Card Electrophysiol 2014;41:203–9.

46. Ricci RP, Morichelli L, Quarta L, et al. Long-term patient Acceptance of and satisfaction with implanted device remote monitoring. Europace 2010;12:674–9.

47. Schoenfeld MH, Compton SJ, Mead RH, et al. Remote monitoring of implantable cardioverter defibrillators: a prospective analysis. Pacing Clin Electrophysiol 2004;27:757–63.

48. Marzegalli M, Lunati M, Landolina M, et al. Remote monitoring of CRT-ICD: the multicenter Italian Care-Link evaluation–ease of use, acceptance, and organizational implications. Pacing Clin Electrophysiol 2008;31:1259–64.

49. Petersen HH, Larsen MCJ, Nielsen OW, et al. Patient satisfaction and suggestions for improvement of remote ICD monitoring. J Interv Card Electrophysiol 2012;34:317–24.

50. Hindricks G, Elsner C, Piorkowski C, et al. Quarterly vs. Yearly clinical follow-up of remotely monitored recipients of prophylactic implantable cardioverter-defibrillators: results of the REFORM trial. Eur Heart J 2014;35:98–105.

51. Morichelli L, Ricci R, Sassi A, Quarta L, Porfili A, al CadedduNet. ICD remote monitoring is well Accepted and easy to use even for elderly. Eur Heart J 2011;32(Suppl. 1):32.

42. Rosenfeld LE, Patel AS, Ajmani VB, et al. Compliance with remote monitoring of ICDS/CRTDS in a real-world population. Pacing Clin Electrophysiol 2014;37:820–7.

43. Ghosh A, Gupta R, Misra A. Telemedicine for diabetes care in India during COVID19 pandemic and national lockdown period: guidelines for physicians. Diabetes Metab Syndr Clin Res Rev 2020;14:273–6.

44. Zhai Y-K, Zhu W-J, Cai Y-L, et al. Clinical- and cost-effectiveness of telemedicine in type 2 diabetes mellitus: a systematic review and meta-analysis. Medicine (Baltimore) 2014;93:e312.

45. Peters AL, Garg SK. The silver lining to COVID-19: avoiding diabetic ketoacidosis admissions with telehealth. Diabetes Technology Ther 2020;22:449–53.

46. Majersik JJ, Reddy VK. Acute neurology during the COVID-19 pandemic: supporting the front line. Neurology 2020;94:1055–7.

47. Velayati F, Ayatollahi H, Hemmat M. A systematic review of the effectiveness of telerehabilitation interventions for therapeutic purposes in the elderly. Methods Inf Med 2020;59:104–9.

48. Zanaboni P, Landolina M, Marzegalli M, et al. Cost-utility analysis of the EVOLVO study on remote monitoring for heart failure patients with implantable defibrillators: randomized controlled trial. J Med Internet Res 2013;15:e106.

49. Guédon-Moreau L, Lacroix D, Sadoul N, et al. ECOST trial Investigators costs of remote monitoring vs. Ambulatory follow-Ups of implanted cardioverter defibrillators in the Randomized ECOST study. Europace 2014;16:1181–8.

50. Ricci RP, Vicentini A, D'Onofrio A, et al. Economic analysis of remote monitoring of cardiac implantable electronic devices: results of the health economics evaluation registry for remote follow-up (TARIFF) study. Heart Rhythm 2017;14:50–7.

51. Heidbuchel H, Hindricks G, Broadhurst P, et al. EuroEco (European health economic trial on home monitoring in ICD patients): a provider perspective in five european countries on costs and net financial impact of follow-up with or without remote monitoring. Eur Heart J 2015;36:158–69.

52. Udwadia ZF, Raju RS. How to protect the protectors: 10 lessons to learn for doctors fighting the COVID-19 Coronavirus. Med J Armed Forces India 2020; 76:128–31.

53. Hindricks G, Varma N, Kacet S, et al. Daily remote monitoring of implantable cardioverter-defibrillators: Insights from the Pooled patient-level data from three Randomized Controlled trials (IN-TIME, ECOST, TRUST). Eur Heart J 2017;38:1749–55.

54. Slotwiner DJ, Abraham RL, Al-Khatib SM, et al. HRS white paper on interoperability of data from cardiac implantable electronic devices (CIEDs). Heart Rhythm 2019;16:e107–27. https://doi.org/10.1016/j.hrthm.2019.05.002.